DATE DUE

2000			

Writing and Getting Published

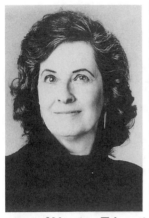

Barbara Stevens Barnum, RN, PhD, FAAN, is Penzance Grant consultant/editor to the Nursing Division, Columbia Presbyterian Medical Center, New York City and editor, *Nursing Leadership Forum* at Springer Publishing Company. Prior to these appointments, she was editor of *Nursing & Health Care*, the journal of the National League for Nursing. Dr. Barnum was Director, Division of Health Services, Sciences and Education at Teachers College, Columbia University, also holding the Stewart Chair in the Department of Nursing Education, and, for part of her tenure, the Chairmanship of the Department of Nursing Education.

Before coming to New York, Dr. Barnum coordinated the Nursing Service Administration Program of the College of Nursing, University of Illinois in Chicago. She also served as Director of Nursing Staff Development at the University of Chicago Hospitals and Clinics. Positions prior to that appointment included chief executive positions in both nursing practice and nursing education at Augustana Hospital and Health Care Center in Chicago.

Dr. Barnum has written widely in areas of nursing management, theory, and education. Her books include *The Nurse as Executive*; *Nursing Theory—Analysis, Application, Evaluation*; and *First-Line Patient Care Management*. Other publications include numerous articles, book chapters, and monographs. She is a Fellow in the American Academy of Nursing and has done extensive national and international consultation and continuing education, including an eight-year term as consultant to the Air Force Surgeon General.

WRITING AND GETTING PUBLISHED

A PRIMER FOR NURSES

Barbara Stevens Barnum
RN, PhD, FAAN

 Springer Publishing Company

An earlier version of this book was published under the Penzance grant, The Presbyterian Hospital of the City of New York.

Springer Publishing Company, Inc.
536 Broadway
New York, NY 10012-3955

Cover and interior design by Tom Yabut
Production Editor: Pamela Ritzer

95 96 97 98 99 / 5 4 3 2 1

Library of Congress Cataloging-in-Publication Data
Barnum, Barbara Stevens.
    Writing and getting published : a primer for nurses / Barbara Stevens Barnum.
        p.   cm.
    Includes bibliographical references and index.
    ISBN 0-8261-8690-4
    1. Nursing—Authorship.   2. Nursing literture—Marketing.
I. Title.
RT24.B37   1995
808'06661—dc20   94-43634
                                                              CIP

Printed in the United States of America

Contents

v

Preface

This book is designed to help the nurse improve her professional writing skills and to help her navigate the publication process. Many a nurse has a great idea for an article or book, but often that is as far as it goes. This book will assist her in getting that article or book off the back burner and into print. The nurse is likely to find this achievement one of the most rewarding in her career.

Of course, there may be many reasons why she does not proceed beyond good intentions in professional writing. Much discomfort with writing can be traced to a nurse's educational program. Crammed with necessary nursing knowledge, her curriculum may have offered few opportunities for honing writing skills. Objective tests were the norm; she was seldom challenged to express herself in essays. After graduation, a demanding job turned her attention to matters of hands-on care.

Yet writing effectiveness is essential for the nurse who wishes to progress in her career. Nurse leaders communicate; indeed, one could argue that writing and speaking skills are what makes them leaders. Effective communication skills are required if one wants to have influence beyond one's immediate circle of friends.

This book is designed to eliminate some of the more common obstacles to effective writing. Contrary to what the nurse may think, the level of writing required in professional communicaions is not complex. After she acquires a few basic skills, the nurse will no longer be inhibited from communicating her ideas in writing.

It is possible for the nurse to have a personally rewarding career without ever writing, but the ability to communicate with one's peers across the nation empowers the nurse, exponentially increasing her influence. This book makes the writing task easier, giving the nurse basic advice on how to write that article or book in a format and fashion likely to meet with a prospective publisher's approval.

The book also tells the writer what to expect between the time an article or book is submitted and when it comes out in print. Often, demystifying the publishing process is all it takes to get a would-be writer started.

Communicating is an important part of the professional nursing role. Vital nursing knowledge is lost when the nurse fails to share her unique insights and discoveries. Other nurses are forced to learn the same facts the hard way simply because her knowledge wasn't placed in the common nursing domain.

The extensive increase in the number of nursing journals in the last few decades testifies that more manuscripts are available than in prior eras. Obviously, many nurses now recognize their obligation to share knowledge and expertise. The large number of journals now in print opens opportunities for the new writer and presents a unique set of choices and problems as well. This book will help the nurse find her way through the maze.

The new nurse writer who wishes to "start big" with a book also has an advantage over professionals in many other disciplines. Publishers are very interested in good nursing books because nurses are known to be avid purchasers. Still other publishers look for good nursing books because of a real commitment to the profession. This is good news to the new writer. If a nurse writes a book with the "right stuff," she will find a publisher, even if she has not yet established her name in the professional literature.

Most new writers prefer to warm up on articles, but it is not unknown for an author to jump right in and start with a book. I can think of several faculty members, for example, who were moved to write because they couldn't find a text that fit a course they wanted to teach. I think of others who were so successful in teaching a course that they wanted to share their content with other educators.

Not that all nursing books need be texts. Effective practicing nurses are great readers too. The nursing field changes rapidly; a committed professional must keep up. And problems faced in the practice setting send nurses seeking solutions in print.

A final word for my male readers: It's always hard, given the limitations of our English language, to decide what rules of grammar should be used regarding sexism. Alas, I've never been comfortable substituting the plural, non-sexist pronouns where I'm really speaking in the singular. That leaves me only the option of selecting a gender-based labelling system. And, personally, I can't stand those articles and books that vary the gender with every paragraph. As a final solution I elected to write this book in the feminine simply because the overwhelming number of people in our profession are women.

I know that men in nursing have had to face this problem over and over, and here I am, asking you to confront it once again. Thanks for your understanding.

Barbara Stevens Barnum, RN, PhD, FAAN

Part I

Writing the Article

Chapter 1

Finding the Right Topic

Writing an article can be a lot simpler than the beginner suspects. The clues given in this chapter will help the nurse organize her article like an experienced writer, in a format most likely to be accepted for publication. But before tackling the nuts and bolts of the writing task, we will examine the motivation for writing in the first place.

COMMUNICATING A MESSAGE

The best reason for writing is that the nurse has something of value to say, something that ought to be shared, something that she truly wants to say. It is best if an idea pushes the writing, not vice versa.

If the nurse has something to say, the writing aspect can be learned. But without an important message, no amount of slick syntax will suffice. Having something to communicate is the first step in successful professional writing.

Having a Position, Not a Subject

When it comes to writing, the nurse needs to communicate specific ideas, not broad generalities concerning subject matters. If she perceives the task as conveying a subject matter, she is likely to talk around a topic broadly, which is never a good idea in an article. Instead, an article hones in on a clear, delimited position. The target of a well-written article usually can be captured in a single sentence. The nurse may benefit from figuring it out and then taping that sentence to the top of her computer where it can serve to keep her focused.

An important difference between subject matter and position is that subject matter is directionless (like *coronary nursing care*), whereas a position is directional. The subject of coronary nursing care does not give any indication what the writer has in mind.

A position, conversely, might be something like the following: "Forced bed rest costs the coronary patient more energy that it saves." Now the writer knows where she is going, and so will the reader.

By a position, I mean something that explains what should happen, what the author recommends. It tells the reader what to do, how to approach a problem, how to analyze a situation. It is pragmatic, with the potential for influencing the way a reader practices in the future.

A position need not be cast against an alternative (for example, bed rest versus no bed rest), although such contrast is a great option for the new writer. Nothing will catch an editor's eye quicker than an article that offers an alternative to accepted ways of doing things. Casting stones at the sacred cows of practice is the meat of which reader interest is made. Look, for example, at these proposed titles for articles:

I Teach My Patients to Be Dependent
Nursing Care Plans: Who Needs Them?
A Good Nurses' Aide Can Be an Effective Primary Nurse

Whether these titles bring a secret smile to a reader's lip or arouse her indignation, could she resist reading the articles? Unlikely. The same is true for the editor who receives such manuscripts.

Yet not all positions need to be *against* something. An effective position paper might offer a way of dealing with a problem that was previously unrecognized as a problem. The idea with a position paper is that it offers some advocacy, suggests some path to be followed. Although a particular subject may be lifeless, a position paper involves the reader (and the editor) immediately, whether she agrees or disagrees with the stance taken.

This is not to say that a position paper is the only kind of article one can write. One of the most interesting articles I've read in the last few years was one in which a nurse searched for the reason why a particular patient on home dialysis got repeated yeast infections. It was a mystery plot, not a position paper, and who can resist a good mystery?

What if the writer has an exciting idea that does not involve a position? Should she drop it? Certainly not. If an idea is exciting, it will make good reading whatever its format. The first prerequisite for a new writer, then, is to have something exciting to say. With an important message, the new writer is halfway home.

The Writer With a Cause

Having said that holding a position was important for a writer, I need to issue a warning. Sometimes a nurse is led to write because she feels so strongly on an issue that she must speak out. This writer starts with a position and a fire in the belly. She may have zeal for her position or anger for those who oppose it. Either way, she is in danger of writing a diatribe instead of an article.

My rule of thumb is that the stronger one feels about a topic, the more restraint one needs in writing about it. No article will sell on the basis of emotion alone. As a matter of fact, unrestrained emotion just does not wash in print. The reader becomes suspect and resistant even if she supports the author's position.

When the writer's emotions are heavily invested in her topic, then more evidence and dispassionate reasoning are required. More passion must be balanced with additional support of one's position. Scathing words will not bring down an opponent nearly as effectively as solid evidence. Moreover, most editors will not touch invective with a 10-foot pole.

Warnings aside, I still recommend the position paper for a new writer because it provides instant interest for the reader, an easy guide for the writing process, and a clear direction that is likely to lead to acceptance by a publisher. An idea presented as a position not only narrows the topic but provides a structure for the article.

If the researcher is dismayed by this recommendation, do not worry. The research article is an exception to the rule; it starts with a question, not a position. Fortunately, the research report has its own ritual reporting structure—a format that, like a position, gives the new writer an easy crutch for the writing process.

FINDING THE RIGHT IDEA

Although it is best to start writing with a burning desire to communicate a message, it is not wrong to view writing as a way to achieve secondary gains—for example, salary perquisites, the acquisition of tenure, or a promotion. A nurse who wants to write for these reasons may not have found her message yet, but that does not mean she lacks one. If the pressure of an upcoming promotion decision provides the impetus, that is fine. Once a nurse gets a push, she often discovers that she possesses valuable information to share.

True, starting in a vacuum, searching for an idea, is a tough way to write. Every nurse remembers the agony of groping for term paper topics in school. Fortunately, there are effective ways for the practicing nurse to find the right idea. This is where her own professional experience and acquired know-how come to the rescue.

Unlike school assignments, the nurse should not pick a topic for an article from a hat. Indeed, her search for an idea should continue until she finds *something to say that is both new and mean-ingful.* That does not mean she must discover an entirely new domain of practice. The uniqueness of her idea may consist of a new way of organizing or perceiving something old and well known.

The best place to look for an idea is the area of practice the nurse knows best. Often the nurse is more of an expert than she realizes, and the first step in writing is to keep a thoughtful eye open as she goes about her practice. Nurses often create effective patterns of practice without recognizing the fact. As she works, the nurse should ask herself:

- What systems, tricks, shortcuts, and safety guards do I recommend to peers?
- What problems have I successfully resolved in nursing situations?
- In what aspects of my work am I particularly expert?

A nurse does not need to write about her particular role, however. It may be special knowledge rather than role performance that provides her unique niche. Has she, for example, been thinking for years about how working in her garden makes her a better nurse? Has she found an effective way to deal with the bullies in her son's kindergarten class? Does she think it might work equally well with drug abusers? Has her class on interior decorating given her insights into some aspect of nursing? Sometimes nonnursing interests stimulate creative thinking about one's profession.

Sometimes the source is more intellectual. Does she have a unique fund of knowledge? For example, has she read every article about left-handedness for years? Does she have an idea how that knowledge might be useful to nurses?

Every day, nurses fail to give themselves credit for their knowledge and expertise. The nurse may assume that if she reasoned something out, everyone else must already know it. Often this is false humility. If a nurse has reached some conclusion, it may well be that others are still puzzled, searching for a strategy, or simply stuck on the problem. The nurse in this situation has found her topic.

The best place to look for a topic is not in a library. A library offers too many distractions, a surfeit of options. The plethora of ideas in a library is overwhelming. Besides, this resource only tells the nurse what has already been written. There is a time for research, but not at the beginning of a writing project, not when the nurse does not yet have her topic.

I suggest that the nurse find a quiet place (a darkened room offers fewer distractions). She should grab a patch of uninterrupted time (children not allowed) and consider those elements of practice that give her the greatest satisfaction, those aspects of her role in which she feels competent. I suggest that she mull these aspects at leisure. She is unlikely to succeed if there is a small imp at the back of her mind saying she has 5 minutes to pick a topic.

Let us consider the nurse who wants to draw on her practice experience. First, she should think about her work as separate from the notion of an article. Let the ideas flow, then a topic will suggest itself. The nurse should write when she has:

- An idea no one else has voiced
- A solution no one else has applied
- A fresh perspective on an old problem
- A new problem no one else has recognized

Whatever the source, the nurse should not stop looking for a topic until she finds one that truly excites her. Writing an article on a topic about which one is indifferent is tough going. An inherent interest, a love of one's subject, is necessary to carry a new writer through the writing process.

Once the writer has her idea, her position, then it is time to research the topic in the library, to make sure her notion is original.

WHAT NOT TO WRITE

Just as it is important to find one's preferred topic, it is also important to make sure the topic is not already overworked. Even if it is near to one's heart, the overworked topic has little chance of acceptance unless the writer really has something different to say about it. A good article, in this case, is not good enough.

Topics that have been overworked in nursing might include decentralization, delegating authority, or using behavioral objectives. Clinical topics do not get to be old hat if the related research or care practices have changed. Still, a "run-of-the-mill" article on the care of a patient having a stroke won't have much chance of publication. Every article should have something new to contribute. If a writer's article is not fresh, she can bet her competitor's article will be.

An overworked topic can be revitalized if the writer's suggestions run against the tide of accepted opinion, present new state-of-the-art information, or provide an entirely new perspective. Such an article is certain to increase the journal's circulation and bring a heavy influx of letters from readers.

How does a writer find out what has been overwritten? Now it is time for that trip to the library. She should check all the journals published in the last few years that are likely to carry the topic of her choice. If the writer is not certain which journals qualify, she needs to get more familiar with the literature. Appendix A of this book lists common nursing journals; sometimes the name of the journal is one's first clue.

This self-directed education will be an interesting exercise. A nurse who has been out of school for a few years will be surprised by the number of new journals in print. The age of the specialty journal has arrived in nursing.

A writer cannot always know what has been overwritten merely by perusing the recent journals. A topic that has yet to reach the library's shelf may be examined in manuscripts presently under preparation at various journals. Because it takes 6 months to 2 years for an article to move through the process from submission to publication, a topic can be overworked before a reader sees a single article on the subject.

If one's topic passes the first test (it does not appear in any recent journals), it is time for query letters to potential editors. This is how the writer learns if her topic is actually timely or dated. See chapter 6 to learn how to write the query letter.

SUMMARY

Picking the right topic is the most important factor in enhancing one's chances for success. The writer must *want* to write the article, and that means she must have a real interest in the topic. Second, she must know the topic thoroughly, usually through a combination of experience and research. Then, in most cases, she needs a viewpoint, a position taken on the subject matter, and, finally, she must have something new to say about the subject, something to catch both the editor's and the reader's eye.

BIBLIOGRAPHY

Diers, D. (1981, spring). Why write? Why publish? *Image, 13*, 308.
Heery, K. (1991, September/October). Who me? Write? *Imprint, 37*, 103–104.
Kilby, S. (1991, January). Write for publication? Who, Me? *The American Nurse*, 30.

Chapter 2

Writing the Article

M any new writers delay communicating important information simply because the notion of writing intimidates them. Yet the structure of the average article is not mysterious. Indeed, there is a simple formula that may be followed. If the writer's material does not fit the formula, however, the reader should feel free to vary from it. The material in this chapter, then, is not given as an absolute set of rules but as a guideline.

SHAPE OF AN ARTICLE

The average article has a classic shape, one that is easy for the reader to follow and easy for the new writer to comprehend. An example follows:

- Dogs like cats (the *one* main point or position to be made).
- My dog Sammy rescued a cat from a burning building (support).
- My neighbor's dog, Fido, sleeps with three kittens (more support).

- The only dog I know who hated cats was taken away for rabies (negative support).
- So you can see, dogs like cats (conclusion).
- I have just told you that dogs like cats, and I have given you evidence: Sammy, Fido, and the rabid dog (summary).

Simple as this structure appears, it is a winning format. The writer makes her point in the first paragraph, then makes sure every subsequent paragraph gives evidence to the same point. This goes on until she thinks she has proved her point, whereupon she states the conclusion. The conclusion, of course, restates her original position. Finally, the article is polished off with a summary.

Notice that the beginning point and the conclusion are identical; one starts and finishes on the same note. On the whole, articles are not mysteries. They move in the opposite direction, starting out with *whodunit*, that is, leading off with a conclusion and supporting it with the rest of the article.

The reader is not kept in the dark. The writer, certainly the inexperienced writer, should tell whodunit at the start. This is not to say that an interesting article cannot be organized as a mystery, but it takes an experienced writer to bring off such a structure.

As the article proceeds through the supporting evidence, it does not hurt to remind the reader periodically of where the article is going by gently reinserting the initial position statement. The writer will want to use slightly different wording each time; if the reader missed the point in one form, she may get it with the restatement.

The number of supporting arguments required will depend on the complexity of the point to be proved. In our example three illustrations were used: Sammy and Fido as positive cases, the rabid dog as negative evidence.

The reader may wish to consider what counts as evidence in supporting arguments. In our simplistic example concerning dogs and cats, only one sort of evidence was offered: personal observation. In professional writing, there are many sources of convincing evidence.

- Personal examples and experiences
- Statistics
- Research findings
- Opinions of experts
- Logical arguments
- Examples from third parties
- Hypothetical cases
- Examples of the predicaments that occurred when the writer's advice was not followed

It has been my experience as an editor that new writers often err on the side of using only one source, usually the opinions of experts. For most articles, the wider the diversity of evidence, the more convincing the argument.

If there is an obvious rebuttal to the writer's position, it does no good to avoid discussing it incidentally. Part of the supporting evidence will have to confront and defeat this alternative position. If the writer does not see any obvious alternative positions, she might ask a friend to play devil's advocate. The simple fact is that if there is another way to interpret her evidence, the writer has to find and deal with this viewpoint.

In addition to presenting ample evidence, the supporting arguments must bear directly on the writer's point. Otherwise, the reader will not accept the conclusion. The best conclusion is the one that *follows* the reader's own intellectual grasp. If the conclusion is premature the reader will not buy it.

The summary follows the conclusion, restates the theme again, and reminds the reader of the main points that have been made. No new information is given at this time. Although the inexperienced writer may feel that the summary is redundant, she must remember that the content is new to her reader. A well-designed summary helps solidify the material in the reader's mind.

To this basic formula of statement, support, conclusion, and summary (restatement), one need only add glue and signposts.

Holding the Article Together With Glue

By glue, I mean the transitions from paragraph to paragraph, section to section. These are the transitional sentences that lead the reader gently from one idea to the next, showing the relationship or the progression.

Let us return to our simple example to see how this works. Two of the supporting themes were:

- My dog, Sammy, rescued a cat from a burning building.
- My neighbor's dog, Fido, sleeps with three kittens.

The connection between these two points may be self-evident to the writer, but the reader should be eased into the second point. The transition sentence or sentences usually come at the beginning of the paragraph introducing a new point. Our example might look something like the following:

> . . . After Sammy's brave rescue of Tiffany, he even carried her home and tucked her into his own doggie bed.
>
> *Sammy may be more heroic than the ordinary dog, but even ordinary dogs get along with cats all the time. My neighbor's dog, Fido, for example, would never be a hero,* but he sleeps with three kittens every night—that is more than their mother Mouser is willing to do.

Adding glue (like the preceding italicized sentences) helps the writer make the leap from one idea to the next. It also helps the writer as much as it helps the reader. In this example, we can imagine that only in searching for the appropriate linking sentences did the writer notice that her examples were different—one about heroic behavior, the other about a nonstressful situation.

Transitional glue makes an article flow. It enables the reader to concentrate on the meaning rather than on the structure of the article.

There are at least two ways to outline an article, and the personality of the writer may determine which is best: forward planning or backward reorganizing.

Who's on First?

There! Did you feel it? That last paragraph about outlines descended on the reader out of the blue. One minute she was reading about transitional glue, then suddenly her thought process was sidetracked by a discussion of outlines. This was not a minor shift—like from Sammy to Fido—this was a major new topic. If the reader felt confused it would not be surprising: the transitional glue was lacking. This is the perfect example of what *not* to do.

Signposts Along the Way

When transitional glue is not strong enough to make the connection between parts of an article, then what is needed is a signpost, a signal to the reader that a new topic will be addressed. The best way to signal a major change in direction is to insert a title or subtitle. We did it here when we switched from transitional glue to signposts.

Most articles, incidentally, try to keep it simple—main topics and perhaps a few secondary subtopics. The content will dictate the appropriate number of levels. Do not use signposts where transitions glue will do. Now and then a writer may need to use a third subdivision, but remember: signposts are designed to make things easier to understand, not more complex.

Now we are ready to use another signpost in *this* chapter; we are about to switch topics again. The new topic will be outlining. If the new topic is part of the main topic already under discussion, it merits a second-level heading (usually positioned at the side). If it is a new topic, it merits a first-level heading (usually centered). In the case of outlining, I think it is outside the scope of the first topic (the shape of an article), so we will make it a first-level signpost.

TO OUTLINE OR NOT TO OUTLINE

I believe there are two kinds of writers: those who will be helped by an outline and those who will be hindered by it, if not downright stopped in their tracks. Perhaps it goes back to that seventh-grade teacher who demanded outlines for every term paper. Every article must be organized, but a formal outline is only one tactic among others.

For those who work best by planning ahead, an outline is ideal. Nor does it have to have the correct labeling: loosely defined topics and subtopics will serve the purpose (so much for the seventh-grade teacher). Those who work with an outline do most of their struggling in getting the outline just right, then they just "fill in the blanks" for the rest of the writing.

Any writing has two parts: discipline and creativity. I suspect that those who start with an outline are simply more comfortable with the first aspect. There are some people who forget what they want to say (the creativity part), however, if it is immediately subjugated to the discipline of an outline. Such a writer does better to just get her ideas down on paper (or computer screen) without giving sequence a thought. After the ideas stop coming, this writer can begin the task of rearranging parts in some logical sequence.

In the era of the typewriter, outlining saved a lot of rewrite time, but in the day of computers, reordering pieces is as simple as "block and move" or "cut and paste," depending on your particular computer's lingo.

FORMATS TO AVOID

Although the writer need not follow the presented format rigidly, there are two kinds of articles that do not fit the format because of their structure. The first one, the unfocused article, fails to fit because it lacks direction. This article has little chance of publication. The second type, the summary article, also has little chance of publication if it offers nothing new.

Actually, there is a third article that does not fit the basic format: the research report. We will not discuss the research report here because it has a unique format that is only a mistake if it is sent to the wrong journal. More about that in chapter 14. For now we will stick to those maverick articles whose formats are mistakes.

Unfocused Article

An unfocused article is one without a real position. Imagine an article on decision making divided into the following segments:

- Decision making: what five authors said about it
- What I tried at work
- Decision making in nursing versus in business
- Difference between decision making and problem solving

This article has a subject matter all right (decision making), but it lacks focus. Four themes are *not* better than one in an article. If a new writer finds her article taking this form, she must consider whether several of her points might be carefully subordinated to serve a main theme. Aspects that cannot be made to serve such a purpose need to be dropped. The writer should not do too much in a single article.

A reader will not follow when diverse themes are presented.

In the back of her mind, the reader keeps asking, "What's her point?" Not that the reader will ask the question for long. The average reader gives up quickly and leafs ahead to the next article. The focus of an article must be limited and clear to draw in the reader. The author must have a viewpoint, and she cannot keep it a secret.

Although it may be difficult for the new writer, she must learn to throw out everything that does not contribute to the singular viewpoint, no matter how inherently interesting the material may be on its own. As we said earlier in this chapter, a good rule for an article is that it make only one major point, that it start with that point, that every paragraph contribute to that point, and that the article conclude with the point repeated.

Summary Article

The summary article gives the state of the art on some subject matter. For example, a summary article on strategic management might have the following structure:

- Strategic management is popular this year . . .
- Author A says . . .
- Author B says . . .
- Author C says . . .
- The conclusion is that strategic management . . .

In truth this manuscript is a term paper, not an article. Chapter 4 will spell out the difference in these formats in more detail. It is enough for the new writer to know that summary articles almost never get accepted for publication. There is the rare exception, however. If, for example, a writer could demonstrate how all these authors were wrong and then give a totally new perspective on strategic management, she would have a good chance for publication.

If a summary article is to catch an editor's eye, it must have a clever and insightful analysis that leads to new views on the topic.

In general, new writers should avoid summary articles; they demand keen insight and complete familiarity with the subject matter.

Most summary articles fail, not because they misrepresent the works of the authorities, but because they fail to express the viewpoint of the author. If a reader wants to know what the experts think, it makes better sense to go to the writings of the experts. A good summary article always tells us something additional about the subject. In essence, the writer must put herself as well as her knowledge, insights, and opinions into the article. Without that personal contribution, an article is sterile.

New writers have to learn this secret in writing all types of articles: They cannot hide behind the opinions of experts or long authoritative citations from other writers. Viewpoints of others can be used to bolster a writer's own position, but her stance cannot be delivered through someone else's words. The reader wants to know what *this* writer thinks. The summary article is always in danger of relying too heavily on the opinions of others. A writer should assume that the reader already knows what the experts have to say.

AUDIENCE

Before the writer actually puts fingers to a computer keyboard, she must decide on an audience. A writer cannot assume that "one size fits all." The same subject matter must be handled differently when addressing nurse researchers, clinical specialists, lay readers, or medical sociologists, for example.

The effective writer targets an audience and keeps that audience in mind the whole time she is writing. Is she speaking to nurse managers? Head nurses? Staff nurses? New mothers? Hospital administrators? Obstetrical clinicians? One speaks in different tongues to different audiences.

Sometimes the same content can be converted into several articles for different audiences, but the terminology, the approach, and even the viewpoint are bound to be influenced by the characteristics of the audience. The new writer should check every sentence to see if she has kept her focus on the chosen audience. Look at the following paragraphs for subtle but uncomfortable shifts in audience:

> In staffing her unit, the head nurse should try to honor staff preferences. She should not ignore the fact that a happy staff simply works better together. The staff nurse should speak up if she objects to her hours, but she should go to her head nurse with solutions in hand. Instead of demanding every weekend off because she wants to attend church, she might first negotiate with her teammate who likes to ski on Saturdays.

> The nurse administrator can prevent suits by making sure that there are iron-clad policies for hazardous situations. For example, patients are vulnerable when learning crutch walking. The staff nurse should make sure her patient wears sturdy shoes with slip-proof soles before attempting crutch walking.

Did your thought processes get "stopped" in either paragraph? Readers react to switches in audience with discomfort. Often they feel the need to reread such a paragraph even if they cannot identify why. After it happens a second time, the usual reaction is to give up and find something else to read.

FINDING A CRITIC

If writing is not the nurse's strong suit, it is useful to have friends criticize a manuscript under preparation. Two dangers exist in this tactic, however. First, some friends hesitate to offer a sound critique. If a friend, however well intentioned, offers only glowing praise, the writer is wise to seek another critic.

A worse problem occurs when the new writer is unable to take criticism. Conversations like the following often occur:

> *Suzy* (pointing to a particular paragraph): I don't know why
>   you say electrolyte imbalance isn't a patient problem.
> *Writer* (shuffling papers): Look, back here on page five,
>   I already said that a patient problem must be perceived
>   by the patient, not the nurse.

This writer is trying to shift the blame for the confusion to Suzy. Even if the writer is technically correct, it is obvious that Suzy missed the point on page 5. If Suzy missed it, so will others. If a reader is confused, the author should not explain it away by placing the failure on the reader. Instead, she should revise the article in a way that is clearer. After-the-fact explanation just does not work. If a reader missed a point, the writer must assume the responsibility for it.

SUMMARY

This chapter has given the new writer some solid advice on how to begin construction of her article. Good construction will not substitute for a lack of ideas, but it will allow the writer to present her ideas in the best possible fashion.

Understanding the basic structure of an article can change the perceived writing task from overwhelming to manageable. It is true that all the rules presented here can and have been broken in numerous articles. Once a writer is experienced, she develops a sense of when deviations from the pattern are possible or even necessary. But the writer can use the basic format as a model until she reaches that degree of experience and writing prowess.

BIBLIOGRAPHY

Blancett, S. S. (1988). The process and politics of writing for publication. *Clinical Nurse Specialist, 2*, 113–117.

Camilleri, R. (1987, winter). Six ways to write. *Image, 19,* 210–212.

Camilleri, R. (1988, fall). On elegant writing. *Image, 20,* 169–171.

Fondiller, S. H. (1992). *The writer's workbook.* New York: National League for Nursing.

Ouellette, F., & Malek, C. (1991, September/October) Streamlining the paper writing process. *Imprint, 38,* 108–111.

Chapter 3

Avoiding Common Mistakes

In my years as an editor, I developed a good sense of where writers go wrong. This chapter will identify the most common pitfalls and the major flaws that condemn an article before it can be judged on other merits. If the new writer avoids these traps, there is no guarantee she will be published, but at least she will have the opportunity to have her writing judged on the worth of its message. Most of the mistakes discussed in this chapter apply to book writing as well, so if the reader has her eye on a book, keep right on reading.

The following sections of this chapter will be stated in the negative, that is, as mistakes to be avoided. I hope this will emphasize the dangers of these particular errors.

BORING TITLES

The title is the writer's first—and sometimes last—opportunity to capture a reader's interest. One should not lose the opportunity. If the writer can pique the reader's curiosity with a title, she is halfway home.

Short, catchy titles that are descriptive of the content of the article are best in my opinion. But sometimes it is difficult to meet all those criteria in one caption. If a choice must be made among criteria, do not eliminate brevity. Look at these titles taken from recent nursing publications.

> Health Locus of Control and Safety Restraint Attitudes in a Sample of Motor Vehicle Accident Victims
>
> Attitudes of Nurse Managers and Assistant Nurse Managers Toward Chemically Impaired Colleagues
>
> A Nursing Department's Response to Risks Associated With Human Immunodeficiency Virus

It is true that these titles are descriptive; the reader knows what will be discussed. But how many of them are exciting? If the reader is not already interested in these topics, the titles do little to lure her in. Compare the preceding titles to the following:

> The Pizza Connection
>
> Changing How Nurses Spend Their Time
>
> Here There Be Dragons
>
> Holding the Mississippi River in Place and Other Implications for Qualitative Research

Notice that all but one of these titles have sacrificed explanation for interest, piquing the reader's natural curiosity. It is difficult to believe that a reader could restrain from reading the first paragraph of these articles. And, with the exception of the last example, they have captured the reader's interest with very few words.

The writer must be guided by the practice of the given journal, whatever its constraints. But even where a comprehensive explanation is expected in the title, one can strive for brevity.

Do *not* write:

> The best way available for the private practitioner to execute chickens when alone and without lethal instruments.

Do write:

How to wring a chicken's neck.

FAILING TO HOOK THE READER

An article must capture a reader quickly; even after a snappy title, it has about one paragraph in which to do the job. After that, most readers turn to another article—and editors know it. The writer must grab the reader by the collar somewhere in the first two sentences. (Editors call this the hook.) Even the most patient reader will not peruse more than a few paragraphs if the purpose of the article is obscure.

There are many ways to get the reader's interest, but the simplest tactic is for the writer to tell the reader where she is going and then deliver on what is promised. Stating a particular position in the first paragraph fills this purpose. And there is no penalty for being amusing, interesting, and clear while doing it.

Other tactics to hook the reader include setting up a puzzle or mystery, appealing to the reader's self-interest, or threatening a sacred cow. These may be considered shock tactics, and they are likely to work provided they are carried consistently throughout the article. For example, one cannot set up a mystery and then ignore it until the last sentence in the article—or worse, fail to solve it. The reader must see how the article unravels the mystery as it proceeds.

Or the reader must be reminded of her self-interest as the article develops, or the sacred cow must be displayed and properly gored.

HIDDEN ARGUMENTS

Hidden arguments are a common error in first-time articles. In this situation, the writer tries to make her argument by moving from what one authority said to what the next one said, then on to the next. Her assumption is that the ideas of these experts taken together comprise a position. In this way the insecure writer tries to hide behind others, masking her own conclusion among their opinions.

The problems presented by this tactic are dual. First, the reader feels cheated if she doesn't hear what the author has to say on the subject. Second, the conclusion that seems so obvious to the writer does not necessarily emerge for the reader. Again, let us take a simplified example to show the mistake. The inexperienced writer will build an argument like the following:

- John (an authority) says cats are clean.
- Jane (an authority) says dogs get dirty.
- Pat (another authority) says cats are the cleanest animals on earth.
- Sally (another authority) says cats are always licking their fur.

In an article constructed in this fashion, the author may *think* that she has made her point clearly: that cats are clean. Yet the reader will not get a sense of a position asserted and proven. The author's position is hidden among citations of experts. Better the writer had come clean in the following fashion:

- I think cats are the cleanest animals.
- John agrees with me, and so do Pat and Sally.
- Jane proves that dogs are not nearly as clean.
- Therefore, *I* am certain cats are clean.

MISPLACED EMOTIONS

There are several cases in which misplaced emotions doom an article to rejection. The first occurs when the tone of an article is overwhelmingly hostile. Nothing makes an article less believable than when anger, rage, or indignation pour from every page.

This is not to say that a writer cannot write about something that has enraged her or stirred some other strong emotion. It simply means that letting the emotion suffuse the article will not work. If the writer is avidly against practice X, she must be able to explain why practice X is wrong in clear, objective terms. As soon as emotion colors her explanations, they become suspect.

It is ironic, but the more a writer feels emotionally involved in a subject matter or position, the more removed and logical must be her approach in writing about it. Emotions may be used like parsley: just a small amount as garnish, please.

The same points made for the negative case also apply to the situation in which the writer is avidly enthused about some cause, position, or pursuit. Colorful bouquets and resounding plaudits will not substitute for logical support of the position. A glowing recommendation engenders reader suspicion if no objective evidence is offered.

Sometimes positive affect is presented as if it were an argument. I recently read an article that could be broken down into the following sections:

- It is time for feminism to take over nursing.
- Feminism is a theory whose time has come.
- Feminism is good for women.
- Most nurses are women.
- Nursing should use feminist theory.

Each segment of this article was reported with unadulterated adulation for feminism and feminists, but there were no hard facts to support the assertions. Even if each of these positions had been adequately supported, the conclusion (that nursing should adopt feminist theory) would not have been logically supported by the prior points.

LATERAL OBLIQUE

The article using the lateral oblique is even more vulnerable to criticism than the article dominated by emotion. In the lateral oblique move, the author takes a position then talks around it. Often she comes back to her position in the conclusion as if she had proved it, when in fact she has not. The lateral oblique argument looks something like the following:

- Every nurse should own a parakeet.
- Parakeets come in all sorts of colors.
- Parakeets learn to talk easily.
- Parakeets are not messy.
- It is easy to love a parakeet.
- Therefore, every nurse should own a parakeet.

Notice that none of these components tells the reader why a nurse should own a parakeet. Even if the parakeet were proved to be the most amiable pet in the world, none of these subsections says why a *nurse* should own one.

IT IS A SIN TO TELL A LIE

This article promises it will do something, then does not do it. It might be considered a subordinate form of the lateral oblique, but it makes a stronger promise. Sometimes the contents of the article appear to support the position taken, but on close scrutiny, they fail the test of evidence. An argument might go this way.

- Teachers can relate to students better if they socialize after hours.
- We always go out bar hopping with our students on Friday nights.
- We even take some of them into our homes for the summer vacation.
- Therefore, we relate to our students better because we socialize with them.

Notice that the evidence given simply is not adequate to support the position. Nor does it tell what kind of relationship is desired with students in the first place. Sloppy logic underlies this presentation.

COMPENDIUM

The compendium is a presumptuous form related to the survey article. The compendium tells everything that was ever written about a given subject matter—for example, hyperventilation, nerve deafness, and decentralization. The survey article typically concerns itself with who said what, whereas the compendium focuses on the facts and fine points rather than worrying about who asserted them. Both forms share a compulsion to tell all, however.

Almost any editor will say the same thing about an article in the form of a compendium: "Don't send it to me, send it to the *Encyclopedia Britannica*."

THREE-IN-ONE ARTICLE

The three-in-one article is a smaller form of the compendium. Here three or more topics, or even positions, are offered as if they constituted a totality. The problem is that they are never adequately tied together. Hence, the article is not one article but three loosely strung together. The form is like the following:

- Touching is good.
- The best form of therapeutic touch is acupressure.
- Science cannot stand therapeutic touch because it conflicts with the medical model.

By the time the reader gets to the end of this article—if she finishes it—she has no idea where the author was going.

CAUTION: ENGLISH LANGUAGE AHEAD

There are other flaws that doom an article in addition to selecting the wrong format. Some of the flaws are so obvious, they seem to go without saying. Yet in my years as an editor, the mistakes occur with depressing regularity. The faults are simple, requiring little explanation. And many of them include deficits in grammar, syntax, spelling, or word choice.

These errors may seem trivial, but they are serious enough to distract the reader from the content. No matter how important the message, an article is likely to be rejected if the writing is awkward, stilted, or ungrammatical. Fortunately, the answer is easy: keep it simple. Here are a few of the most common errors.

Incomplete Sentences and Incorrect Grammar

Many articles fail to follow the basic rules for forming sentences—namely, that every sentence have a subject and predicate. When a sentence is long and comprised of many complex phrases, the need for a subject and predicate may be forgotten in the rush of words. This alone is a good reason for keeping it simple.

If a writer is insecure about her ability to handle the English language, any freshman-level text on composition will be well worth the price. Many writers use the short and simple book by Strunk and White listed in the bibliography.

Complex Phrasing

A sentence should use the fewest words and the least ostentatious phrasing. *Now* is always preferable to *at this point in time. The machine has parts A, B, and C* is preferable to *the machine is comprised of the component parts A, B, and C.* No editor likes stuffy, pseudoerudite phrasing.

The writer should not use a seven-syllable word if a one-syllable word will do, nor five sentences where one could convey the same message. I call this pretentious form *nursese* because so many nurse writers do it. This affected style always complicates the reader's ability to understand what is being said. Look at the following example:

> *Nursese*: Hypothetically, it is possible that several attempts to alter the water flow may meet with failure before the objective is achieved.
> *English*: You may have to experiment with the water flow before you get it right.

In the same vein, the writer should avoid nursing jargon. The writer should not coin a new word unless she has actually invented a new concept never before used by humankind that is, therefore, unnamed. Most ideas can be expressed adequately in the language already available to the writer. A writer should explore existing options before creating a new lexicon of terms.

Passive Voice and Awkward Sentence Structure

Articles that stick to the active voice have a better chance of publication for two reasons: They are easier to read, and they convey vibrancy and movement. In active voice the subject of the sentence does the acting rather than being acted on by the verb. Compare the following paired sentences:

> Mrs. Jones was kept in doubt about her diagnosis by the physician.
> The physician kept Mrs. Jones in doubt about her diagnosis.

Nursing acts that are difficult to justify under King's theory
of nursing are involved when taking care of an unconscious patient.

Taking care of an unconscious patient involves nursing
acts difficult to justify under King's theory of nursing.

In both cases the second wording is easier to understand. When
the thoughts to be expressed are complex as in the second example,
the active voice is essential.

Avoid complex sentence structure unless there is no alternative. Compare the following two sentences:

After having gotten tangled in the sheets and having fallen
from the bed, the patient fractured his hip.

The patient got tangled in the sheets, fell from the bed,
and fractured his hip.

Honestly, which sentence would anyone rather read?

Illogical Order

If there is a natural order to her material, the writer should use
it. The order in the first draft is seldom the best order, yet reordering is something new writers often forget to do. I once received an article discussing the use of the nursing process that
went like this: After describing the nursing process, the writer
talked about assessment, then nursing diagnosis, followed by
nursing care. Then she had some additional thoughts about
assessment followed by a discussion about evaluation and, finally, a section on new trends in diagnosis. With little work, the
related elements could have been reorganized according to the
steps of the nursing process. As it was, the article felt jumpy,
and her points got lost in all the back-and-forth movement among
elements.

Paragraphs That Do Not Link

As we said in the last chapter, the greatest flaw among new writers is forgetting transitions and signposts. The reader needs clear signals of how what follows links to what came before. Although the error may occur between sentences, it is more likely to occur between paragraphs. Consider the following example in which the first sentence represents the end of one paragraph, the next sentence the beginning of the next paragraph:

> Many new assignment systems are being tested in this age of restructured practice.
> Manthey's concept of paired partners is presently being used in five hospitals in . . .

If this happens to be the first time the reader has heard of paired partners, she may not understand how these two paragraphs link. The writer could have prevented this confusion by saying something like the following:

> Many new assignment systems are being tested in this age of restructured practice.
> Among the new assignment systems, Manthey's concept of paired partners is a popular choice. It is presently being used in five hospitals in . . .

The reader may think I am giving too much space to linkage problems, but in my experience it is the chief flaw of inexperienced writers, *and* it is the flaw most likely to make the editor pitch an article in the circular file.

SUMMARY

A poorly crafted article with a really significant message may be accepted by an editor who has the time and commitment to rewrite it, but that does not happen often in today's publishing world. Let us face it, few ideas are truly earth shaking. But a moderately interesting idea, presented in an orderly and sensible fashion, has a good chance of being published.

With a little care, the writer can avoid the mistakes illustrated in this chapter. Taking the time to eliminate these errors will pay off. It is sad when a flawed presentation prevents a nurse from sharing a really great idea.

The writer cannot afford to underestimate the importance of form and format. It is like preparing a tray for a patient who is not hungry. He may not eat the rose or the parsley garnish, but they help improve his appetite.

BIBLIOGRAPHY

Barzun, J. (1975). *Simple and direct: A rhetoric for writers*. New York: Harper & Row.

Cook, C. K. (1985). *Line by line: How to improve your own writing*. Boston: Houghton Mifflin.

Floren, J. (1989). *Write smarter, not harder*. Wheaton, IL: Twain Productions.

Fondiller, S. H., & Nerone, B. J. (1993). *Health professionals stylebook: Putting your language to work*. New York: National League for Nursing.

Goldensohn, E. (1982). Acute, fulminating jargonitis. *Nursing Outlook, 30*, 541.

Huth, E. J. (1990). *How to write and publish papers in the medical sciences*. Baltimore: Williams & Wilkins.

King, L. S. (1978). *Why not say it clearly: A guide to scientific writing*. Boston: Little, Brown.

McCarty, P. (1991, January). Nurse authors share writing tips. *The American Nurse*, 31–32.

O'Connor, Andrea B. (1976). *Writing for nursing publications*. Thorofare, NJ: Charles B. Slack.

Schlosberg, J. (1994, January). Article-writing blueprint step 3: Raising the rough draft. *Writer's Digest*, 32–35.

Sheridan, D. R., & Dowdney, D. L. (1986). *How to write and publish articles in nursing.* New York: Springer.

Strunk, W. J., & White, E. B. (1979). *The elements of style* (3rd ed.). New York: MacMillan.

Ventura, M. R. (1992). Guidelines for writing for publication. *Journal of the New York State Nurses Association, 23,* 16–19.

Zinsser, W. (1983). *Writing with a word processor.* New York: Harper & Row.

Zinsser, W. (1988). *On writing well* (2nd ed.). New York: Harper & Row.

Zorn, C. R., Smith, M. C., & Werley, H. H. (1991). Watch your language. *Nursing Outlook, 39,* 183–185.

Chapter 4

It's a Great Term Paper: Why Don't You Get It Published?

In graduate study many nurses are encouraged by their instructors to seek publication of excellent term papers, only to be disappointed when these papers are rejected. There are two common reasons why an editor turns down such a paper: (a) It may offer nothing new on the subject matter, or (b) the author may have failed to convert the term paper into article format. The term paper we refer to here is the scholarly work, a researched paper on an assigned or selected subject matter.

PAPER WITH NOTHING NEW TO SAY

An instructor may be duly impressed by a paper demonstrating that a student has full grasp of a subject matter; after all, that is her job—educating students. In contrast, an editor is looking for a paper that contributes something new to the subject. Her position is that if one wants to know what Nurse X said about subject Y, one is better off reading Nurse X's work than perusing someone else's secondhand interpretation of what Nurse X said.

A paper that merely accumulates the wisdom of others has little chance of being published. This sort of paper—we called it a summary article in earlier chapters—will not be published unless it contributes some new content or unique analysis. If it points out where all the experts were wrong, an editor might be interested. If it gives a new or antithetical outlook on their conclusions or explains the limitations of their analyses, it might catch an editor's eye.

In other words, a good scholarly paper that simply accumulates the opinions of experts may please a teacher, but it will bore an editor. One way for a writer to test her paper is to go through it, underlining the opinions and contributions of others in blue, and her own opinions and contributions in red. If there is little red when she is finished, there is little likelihood of publication.

SCHOLARLY PAPER SUBMITTED IN TERM PAPER FORMAT

Suppose that the writer indeed has something new to say in her term paper. She still has to surmount the problem of format. The styles of term paper and article are quite different. An adequate conversion to the appropriate format may make the difference between an acceptance and a rejection.

If the writer already has the subject matter in hand, the research completed and the ideas matured, the conversion process is a minor matter. The following discussion compares the scholarly term paper and the article, providing clues for reorganizing a paper for publication.

1. *A scholarly paper proves the writer knows all there is to know about a given subject matter; an article makes a point.* The scholarly paper cites lots of authors, giving quotations from each. Often this is done to prove the writer's scholarly credibility.

    In contrast, an article never cites an author unless

the quote has a direct bearing on the particular point being made. Quotes are limited and *to the point*. The writer must remember that the reader is not a faculty member; she does not *have* to read the article. And she will only stay with it as long as it is interesting.

A good bibliography at the end of the paper will prove the writer knows the appropriate sources. The bibliography substitutes for the literature review found in a scholarly paper.

2. *A scholarly paper talks broadly about a subject matter; an article takes a position.* For example, a scholarly paper might address "New Baccalaureate Nursing Programs," but a related article might take the position "New Baccalaureate Programs Fail to Prepare Nurses for Practice in the Home Setting."

The difference is critical. A scholarly paper covers a subject in breadth, often "talking around" the topic. In contrast, an article takes a position in relation to some aspect of the topic.

In searching a scholarly paper for a topic for an article, one is likely to find several possibilities. The writer's task is to select one, and subordinate other items in the paper to that idea or eliminate them. The side trips that delight a teacher are distracting in an article. The writer must select the one best focus and stay with it.

The writer can check to see that she has a *position* instead of a *subject matter* by considering these questions: What should be the reader's response after reading this article? What should she do? If the writer can answer these questions, she has achieved the level of specificity required. To say that the reader will simply know more is not adequate.

3. *The writer of an article must stick to the theme; the scholarly paper loves those interesting side trips.* One or two side issues, closely related to one's main position may be retained in an article if they are sub-

ordinated to the main point, but the writer should not tackle too much in a single article.

Scholarly papers diverge; articles converge. More than three major points in an article, and the writer will have lost much of the audience or worse, the potential editor. Each paragraph of an article must work to support the central position. If a paragraph fails this test, it should be removed.

4. *A scholarly paper works up to a conclusion (if any); an article begins with one.* In the scholarly paper, the conclusion is found at the end where everything is pulled together. An article goes in the opposite direction, starting out with a conclusion that is supported or explained in the rest of the manuscript. The reader is not kept in the dark; good articles are rarely mystery stories. A basic structure for an article is captured in the advice: Make your point, support your point, and make your point again.

5. *A scholarly paper does not have to be interesting, only accurate; an article must be both.* As discussed in the last chapter, an article must woo its reader. The writer must keep reader interest in mind at all times.

6. *A new and catchy title will probably be required in converting a scholarly paper to an article.* Again, drawing reader interest is the goal. Notice the title of this chapter. It might have read, "Conversion of a Scholarly Paper to an Article." But the title given was selected for article appeal: "It's a Great Term Paper: Why Don't You Get It Published?"

RETRACTIONS

Having said that journals will not accept term papers, I need to come clean and say that there are a few journals that will accept a scholarly term paper. Often these are journals that mostly publish research reports, fleshing their issues out with nonresearch reports that come as close as possible to research without actually doing it. Some term papers may qualify.

These journals are in the minority, but as I have said before: Match your style with that of the articles already published in the journal. For most journals, an unmodified term paper simply will not do.

SUMMARY

Scholarly papers are not articles, but they are great sources for articles. Mining a good scholarly paper for the buried treasure is great fun and makes the most of the work the writer already did in learning the subject. Conversion is not half as difficult as a new writer anticipates.

Almost every nurse has a good term paper stashed away somewhere in her files. It is not a bad idea to dig it out and see if a great article is hidden there.

BIBLIOGRAPHY

Nurse Author & Editor. (1991). Avoiding the "school paper" style rejection. *Nurse Author & Editor, 1* (3), 1–6.

Chapter 5

Publication Options: Sending Your Article to the Right Journal

Finding the right publisher is almost as important as the writing of an article itself. Making a careful study of the options saves the author time and increases her chances of getting published. If an article grows moldy in the hands of an editor who is not certain the work is for her, the writer has only herself to blame. In all cases, the writer's task is the same: to send her writing to the source or sources most likely to publish her type of material.

SELECTION BY VIRTUE OF THE AUDIENCE

Sometimes an author has a clear idea of the audience she wants to reach. In this case, it is best to select the journal before writing the article. This makes great sense when one considers the vast differences in style and content, for example, between *Redbook* and *Nursing Research*. If the comparison brought a smirk to your lips, think again. Too often nurses ignore the public, nonnursing press. This arrogance means that the public has little idea what nurses do and know.

Writing for the General Public

Suppose a writer decides to write for the public press. If she is a nurse, it is likely that her library at home is stacked mostly with nursing journals (with, perhaps, *The New Yorker* and *Newsweek* creeping in). Obviously, a trip to the local newsstand will be required. The writer will not merely want to browse the racks for likely magazines, but she will want to purchase many general consumer magazines to take home for more intensive inspection.

She will need to study each magazine in detail and ask herself: Who reads this journal? Young women? Older women? Men? What is the average education of the reader? *Savvy* and *Reader's Digest* may cater to people with different levels of education. What are their interests? *Modern Bride* and *Cosmopolitan* might reach a similar age group of women, but their interests will be different.

Selling an article to a journal in the general consumer press is more difficult than getting published in a professional journal. There is more competition for space, and the nurse is competing with people who make their livings as professional writers. Nevertheless, she has a special expertise on which to draw: nursing. A benefit, of course, is that she may gain access to a really large readership. But to sell an idea to any public consumption journal, one has to meet a special interest of the magazine's editor and readers.

The task may be easier if the nurse writer can relate to the intended audience. *Working Woman*? She certainly shares some background with these readers. Is she raising children? Maybe one of the many journals focused around family would be the source for her.

In the public press, having a hook to catch the reader's interest (as well as sustaining it) is even more important than in professional journals. Indeed, you may need a "new twist" to grab the editor's interest at all. But if the public is the best audience for your message, go to it.

One advantage of consumer publications is that they often pay for articles, an added bonus unlikely in a professional journal. Many consumer magazines run health columns, but at present most of them are authored by physicians. There is no reason why an entre-preneurial nurse could not make writing such a column her goal. Consumer magazines about health are becoming more popular, increasing the options for the writing nurse.

Writing for Other Professions

Too often nurses fail to submit relevant articles to nonnursing professional journals. Is the nurse's topic one that might appeal to the *New England Journal of Medicine*? Is the article about medical ethics? Has she considered law journals or journals that focus on ethics? As is the case with the public press, nursing often ignores these viable alternatives. The whole profession benefits when good articles by nurses reach the journals of other professions.

Another advantage of publishing in related professional fields is that an article may be suitable for publication in both nursing and another profession, getting "double mileage" out of one's work. Chapters 8 will discuss the legalities involved in such double publication.

WRITING FOR A SPECIFIC JOURNAL

If a writer is convinced that her article should be published in a particular journal, then all efforts can be directed to that end. First she will intensively study its style; then she can begin writing.

There is a risk in writing for a specific journal. Some, but not all, journals are so unique that an article written for a given outlet will not fit elsewhere. If the writer selects one of these journals, the danger is that, if rejected, she will probably have to start all over, redesigning the article for the next submission.

Sometimes, if the writer is lucky, the only change required will be in format. It is not a good idea, for example, to submit an article to *Nursing & Health Care* with the bibliography in the style required by *Holistic Nursing Practice*. Trust me, one look at the bibliography and, not only will the editor know that the article was rejected elsewhere, but she will even know which journal rejected it.

Sometimes a writer can bridge journals in her mind, writing an article that works best for one journal while still being compatible with the style and content of a second or even a third journal. This possibility is more common in professional writing than in writing for the general public. The worst danger, however, is *not* revising the article if it is sent to a second journal.

As an editor, I often smiled when reading an article that I could *tell* was originally meant for another journal. And when an editor figures out that she is reading an article that has already been rejected elsewhere, need I tell you her first instinct?

Sometimes the choice of whether to begin by writing the article or by selecting the journal is not an either-or option. The two necessities may come together as the writer begins to put her thoughts to paper.

Nevertheless, there are some cases in which the writer is so absorbed with her message that she only thinks about potential journals later. When this happens we are usually talking about an article for the professional nursing press. Let us turn to that case.

SEEKING A JOURNAL FOR A FINISHED ARTICLE

In selecting a journal for an article that has already been written, the writer first must know the nursing literature. Then she must read several recent issues of any journal she is considering. Matching content is the first step. She should not, for example, send a highly clinical article to a journal that deals with the politics of health care and nursing trends. Although this sounds like stating the obvious, I cannot count the times, as an editor, I received materials inappropriate for the content of my journal.

Not only must the subject matter be right for the journal, but the format must be consonant as well. If the journal only publishes research reports, for instance, there is no sense sending an opinion piece. Nor would such a journal accept a how-to article. Nor is a case study likely to be accepted by a journal that has never published one. The writer should pick a journal whose format matches that of her article.

Simply put, the writer should make sure her article sounds like the articles the journal presently is publishing. The other option is to adapt her article to the format of the journal. Either way the match should be made before the manuscript is submitted.

The degree of formality should be a match too. Some journals are folksy; others take a stiff, professional tone. Some like a literary style; others mimic medical journals in their scientific patina.

If the author is in a hurry to get her article to the public, other considerations may come into selecting a journal. On the whole, she can assume that the better-known journals will receive more articles, sometimes slowing down the review process, and often delaying the time between acceptance and publication. In addition, journals that get more submissions can be more selective. The new writer may not be ready for this market.

Specialty journals may be easier targets than the *American Journal of Nursing*, for example. Even better, newer journals may have less of a backlog of accepted articles. Not only may the new writer have a better chance of having her article accepted by a new publication, but it may come out in print sooner.

SUMMARY

Selecting the right journal is essential in getting acceptance for one's article. The writer must be sensitive to how her material fits that which the journal publishes. It does not make sense to waste time soliciting journals where the match simply is not right.

With a little effort and research, the writer can avoid this pitfall and the subsequent disappointment engendered when her material is rejected. The right content in the right style for the right audience: a recipe for success.

BIBLIOGRAPHY

Cosgray, R. E. (1991). I wish I could publish something. *Imprint, 38,* 167–170.

Evans, N. (1981). Authors and publishers: The mutual selection process. *American Journal of Nursing, 81,* 350–352.

Glover, S. M. (1991, January). Getting published: Guidelines for prospective authors. *The American Nurse,* 29.

Huston, C. (1988, spring). A guide to publication for nurses. *Nursing Connections, 1,* 85–91.

Jiminez, S. L. (1991, spring). Consumer journalism: A unique nursing opportunity. *Image, 23,* 47–49.

Chapter 6

What About a Query Letter?

The query letter is a good place to start in getting an article published in a nursing journal. It is essential in dealing with the consumer press. A query letter assists an author in surmounting several obstacles that stand between her and publication, and, equally important, helps her avoid wasting time. A query letter simply asks whether an editor might be interested in an article one plans to write or has already written.

ESSENCE OF THE LETTER

A good query letter gives the working title and a short description of the proposed article. The letter should be skillfully crafted because it gives the editor a sense of one's skill in handling grammar, syntax, and ideas.

The letter not only gives the paper's topic, but its premise and structure as well. The more one tells an editor without getting wordy, the better. Nevertheless, the letter should be limited to one page or two at the most. Longer queries tend to get buried on an editor's desk under other work that can be completed with more efficiency. Those that are succinct get a quick response.

Do not waste space telling the editor how great the article is or how much her journal needs it. Frankly, she will be the judge of that. And she is unlikely to feel positive about an author trying to tell her how to do her job.

The purpose of a query letter is to see if an editor is interested in the subject matter of a proposed article. Query letters may be sent to 1 editor or 20 simultaneously; they do not commit an author to sending the completed article to a given journal.

Nor does an editor's positive response to a query mean that her journal is committed to publication of the final work. A positive response simply means that the editor will give serious consideration to a well-written article on the subject matter. If a writer receives a positive response to the query letter, she should remind the editor of that fact when she submits the final article to that editor.

MECHANICS

Although a crisp description of the proposed article is the essence of the query letter, amenities count. The same rules that apply to submitting a manuscript (see Chapter 7) apply to the query letter. The writer should make sure the letter reaches the right person, addressed by the right name, at the right journal.

The query letter also should contain reference to the writer's credentials, although this may be more important to some editors than to others. For example, a good political piece may be attractive no matter who wrote it, but a clinical piece on a special type of patient care will be bolstered by the author's relevant clinical experience and specialty credentials.

One cannot expect credentials to substitute for a terse, clear description of the article. Nor is it necessary for the author to include a complete copy of her curriculum vitae at this time.

A writer should not send a query letter if she intends to ignore the editor's advice. In other words, it is a waste of time to submit an article to an editor after she's given a negative response to a query letter. Editors have long memories. If the writer has her heart set on submitting the article to journal X, then she might as well wait and send the article directly without giving the editor a chance to reject it in a query.

EDITOR'S RESPONSE

Editors vary in how much time they allot to answering queries. Sometimes the author gets a terse note saying the editor is interested or not interested. Other editors take the time to give reasons.

If comments are received, they should be read carefully, because they often make the difference between a publication and a near miss. Even if the writer ultimately decides to send an article to a different editor, what was a problem for one editor may be a problem for the next one as well.

More important, an editor may suggest a unique perspective or angle to take on the subject matter. When this happens, the writer probably has a good chance at publication if the article can be structured as suggested.

The editor's comments are not dictates, but a writer should consider them seriously unless they go against the essence of her article. Any editor has her own preferences and knows the preferences of her review board. If she is giving a writer a hint, the writer should take advantage of it—even if it means revising an article she hoped was finished.

WHEN YOU ARE REJECTED

Query letters get negative responses for many reasons, not all of which can be predicted. Some factors can be estimated with greater reliability than others. It is not difficult to tell whether a given subject matter is an appropriate fit with a given journal, for example.

Conversely, what appears to be a perfectly good subject matter may not be of interest if the editor has several articles on the same subject already being prepared for publication.

This situation is something a writer cannot know except by query. Unfortunately, from the perspective of the author, what seems to be a fresh idea may not be all that fresh to an editor. Every editor knows that a new idea tends to occur to lots of people in the same time frame. Indeed, it is not surprising for an editor to be swamped with several articles on the same subject matter, even though each author thinks it is a brand new notion.

Moreover, there may be organizational influences—for or against her topic—that an author cannot anticipate. Of course, an author might easily predict that an article condemning nursing school accreditation might not readily be accepted by the journal of the accreditation body. Yet she might not know how welcome her article on grief following loss of a child will be if the journal is about to launch a new column on bereavement. Similarly, an article advocating that we do away with textbooks might get an unwelcome response from a journal published by a book company.

It is not possible for a writer to know all the inside politics and values that affect a given journal. And that is where the query letter saves a lot of time.

A writer should never, incidentally, write a query letter unless she does it properly. A query dashed off on yellow note pad is a certain invitation to rejection. Even if the writer's topic is an interesting one, she has done nothing to convince the editor that she is up to the work of producing a professional article on the subject.

TELEPHONE CALL

Some editors are willing to substitute a telephone call for a query letter. A call can achieve the same objective, provided the editor is willing to operate this way, and provided the author brings all the information to a telephone conversation that would otherwise have been included in a written inquiry.

This means the writer has her points in front of her, on paper, before she picks up the telephone. A telephone conversation is not a substitute for a query letter if the writer has not yet figured out the details of her article. And beware: If the editor has questions, the nurse better be ready to answer them. Suppose the editor asks how her paper compares to the classic work on the subject by Howe. If the nurse has not even heard of Howe, you can bet the editor will not be impressed. The writer who is not good at thinking on her feet may wish to avoid the option of a telephone call.

Conversely, some editors will be more forthcoming in a telephone conversation, taking time to discuss the ways in which such an article might or might not work for her journal. The writer may get more detailed advice on the telephone concerning how to slant the article and how to improve its chances for acceptance.

Not all editors respond to query telephone calls positively. If a writer calls an editor, she should be up front about the purpose of the call, asking first if the editor is willing to discuss a query by telephone. She should indicate her willingness to put the information in writing if the editor prefers.

Conversely, some editors welcome the quick telephone call. After all, it saves them the time involved in composing a response and saves the writer time as well.

WHY QUERY?

The most important function of a query letter is to save the author time. Many query letters can be sent simultaneously, whereas an article should, generally, be submitted to only one journal at a time.

Let us take the worst case scenario: An author skips the query letter and submits an inappropriate article to a journal. Suppose the article is sent out to the review panel. It could take up to 3 months before the panel members respond and the author receives the inevitable rejection. Hence, 3 months have been wasted before the article can be sent to a second journal where it might have a chance for acceptance. A good query letter could have saved 3 months.

A good query letter has another advantage: It forces the author to think out her plan and message for an article. When an author sits down to write the query, she will find the flaws in her conceptualization. In addition, the same precis can form the basis for the article abstract.

SUMMARY

The query letter does not so much insert an extra step in the publication process as streamline it. The time spent in a query can save an author months of wait time. More important, a query letter can make the difference between an acceptance and a rejection. An editor always gives a full reading to an article sent on the basis of her positive response to a query.

Chapter 7

Submitting Articles: Getting the Procedures Right

Sometimes the procedures for formatting and submitting an article discourage a first-time writer. In practical terms, the procedures involve exercising good sense. But the following details should take out the worry, leaving the author free to concentrate on the important part—namely, the content of her article. Now and then an article is lost or misdirected if the proper procedures are not followed, so adhering to them can make a difference.

ACCOMPANYING LETTER

Every article submitted to an editor should be accompanied by a brief letter giving all the identifying information on a single page. The writer should make sure it contains the title of the manuscript, and the full name, address, and telephone number for each author. Authors with their credentials and titles should be listed in the same order as desired if the article is published. If the article is clinical, the writer may wish to include a curriculum vitae for each author.

For other types of articles, vitae may be included but will not be as critical at this time. If the article calls for a unique and special form of expertise, it is important that the editor know the author qualifies.

If several authors are listed, the writer must be clear as to which one is the corresponding author. Usually the article is submitted by this person, but it does not hurt to clarify. Editors usually will not correspond with more than one author during the review/ publication process.

An editor should never be expected to serve as a mediator between or among authors. Coauthors should have reached agreement on all aspects of handling the article before submitting it. If questions come up later—for example, whether a given chart could be omitted—it is up to the corresponding writer to settle that point with her fellow authors, then get back to the editor.

It seems only good sense that the accompanying letter contain the address of the correspondent; however, after serving years as an editor, I know it does not always happen. Remember, secretaries throw away envelopes. Therefore, the writer must put her return address on the letter itself.

For courtesy's sake, she should be sure to address the letter to the present editor. One can find out the editor's name by looking at the front matter of the *latest* issue. Do not trust a journal copy from last year; editors move around a lot.

Sometimes there are several editors for a journal, and the writer may be confused over which one should be addressed. A rule of thumb is that the editor or editor in chief is more likely to be the appropriate target than the managing editor. Normally the managing editor tends to production details, whereas the editor makes content decisions.

One cannot count on this, however, and two separate journals may have different job descriptions for people with the same title. If the article reaches the wrong editor, it is likely to be forwarded to the correct person. But the writer may lose time at best, and, at worst, her article may be misplaced.

When in doubt, the writer can take the simple expedient of calling the editorial offices of the journal. The secretary will be pleased to give the proper editor's correct name and mailing address.

When last I managed a journal that had had prior editors, I often received correspondence directed to an editor who had preceded me by 15 years. Although this never caused me to turn down an excellent article, I looked with a jaded eye if the subject matter of the submitted article required the author to be on top of trends. To fail to use the editor's name shows a certain carelessness that she will not appreciate. And it reveals you as a rank amateur—not an impression designed to produce a positive response.

Nor should the writer be lazy and skip the editor's name. A letter addressed to "Dear Editor" will travel directly to the wastebasket in many editorial offices.

FORMAT FOR THE ARTICLE ITSELF

Almost every journal has an author's guide. It simplifies things if the author will write for a copy of this information while her article is in process. Following these directions allows the writer to tailor the article to the journal.

Conversely, most editors will not disqualify a good article if it deviates in minor ways from the guidelines. For example, suppose that the author used a common citation system that differed from the journal's style. Most editors will read such a paper; some few may require it be changed before sending it out to reviewers. If an editor accepts an article that deviates from the format used, she will probably ask the author to revise it. Some few will even let a copy editor make the appropriate changes.

Main Text

Because an article should only be sent to one journal at a time, a writer really has little excuse for not adopting the preferred style from the start. If an article comes in a different format, the editor may wonder if it were written for another journal first, then sent along to her when it was rejected. Such a suspicion is unlikely to turn off acceptance of a really top-grade article; however, in borderline cases, impressions may weigh more heavily.

At the present time far more articles are written in the nursing field than possibly can be published. Therefore, it is not simply a question of whether an article is worthy of publication but of whether it is *more* worthy than the other available papers at the time.

Given the competition, there is no use creating unnecessary obstacles. Ideally, a writer wants her article considered on the merits of its content. The following material will give the standards followed by most editors. If a journal's guide differs from these, the writer should follow the supplied guide.

The cover page should include the title, authors in preferred order, their credentials and titles, and their telephone numbers and mailing addresses. Today some authors include fax numbers. Even though the editor will normally correspond with only one author, there are often emergencies when an editor is glad to have the other contact information in her files.

Other front matter includes an abstract and key words. The *abstract* should be the length printed in that journal. A writer should not send a two-page abstract to a journal that prints a single paragraph (the common size). Sending an abstract does not ensure that an editor will use it; she may prefer to make up her own if the article is published. But whether she uses the supplied abstract or writes her own, she will appreciate having a copy from which to work.

In those rare cases where abstracts are not printed in a journal, send one anyway. They may be used for other purposes inhouse. If there are no guidelines, keep it terse—a few paragraphs.

Key words are the titles (usually one or two words each) by which the author wants the article referenced in printed indexes and in the various computer on-line retrieval systems. The writer need not worry if she is unfamiliar with the titles used in each system. She can simply select the five or six captions (common terminology please) that make the most sense, that is, those titles that best capture the subject matter of the article. If they are not suitable, the indexer will select other titles. As with the abstract, the writer's suggestions will be appreciated but not necessarily used.

Related Matter

How many copies should be submitted? Four or five copies of the article will suffice if the journal is refereed or if the writer is uncertain of the procedures to be followed.

Most professional journals are refereed these days, and that is to the writer's advantage. A refereed journal is one that selects articles based on the advice received from a panel of experts versed in the subject matter of the paper. Some colleges and universities do not count publications in unrefereed journals when making tenure decisions. For a faculty member, finding out whether a journal is refereed may be a critical factor.

In the past, most journals required *an original* and a given number of copies. This was to emphasize that articles go only to one source at a time. In today's world, there is no need for an original unless the article was typewritten. Today, most articles (I would guess about 95%) are computer generated, making the question of originals irrelevant.

If the author does send photocopies, she should make sure to have clear, clean copies. Editors spend most of their waking hours reading, and they do not appreciate receiving difficult-to-read copies. Never, incidentally, send a manuscript printed on dot matrix. Most editors simply will not subject themselves to the eye strain.

A writer need not send a computer disk of an article until it is accepted. Indeed, the article may go through several revisions in the interim. Reviewers and editors may make valuable suggestions the writer may wish to incorporate in the final version.

Computer disks almost never are returned, and the writer should submit only one—the final version before in-house copy editing. Nothing is more frustrating to an editor than to discover she has two disks on file, one likely obsolete. Extra steps, such as determining which is which, are not appreciated by the typesetter either.

Almost all editors prefer the same *format for pages*: double-spaced, on a single side of nonerasable white paper. Paginate, please. Editors' offices are messy; manuscripts cover not only an editor's desk but every available surface. Briefcases overflow too, and pages can get separated accidentally. I admit there may be one or two extremely neat editors, but I have not met them yet. If an article gets out of order, the editor may not be in the mood to figure out the right sequence. So protect your manuscript: Paginate.

The upper right corner is a convenient spot for page numbers unless the guidelines differ. For extra protection, it is convenient if the first author's name appears on the left-hand side of every page, across from the page number. It goes without saying that colored paper is difficult to photocopy and should not be used.

Although articles may look more interesting when printed with diverse *fonts* (*typefaces* in the case of typewriters), to submit an article in this form is the sign of an amateur. Use only one font, preferably the plainest, most legible one available. The writer should underline rather than use italics.

As to *length*, in most journals the average article runs about 15 typewritten/computer-printed, double-spaced pages. One may have problems getting an article accepted if it deviates much from that standard. Incidentally, editors calculate these things far more often than do authors, so a paper that is single spaced or printed in an elite type in an attempt to decrease the page count, does not fool anyone.

Unless the article of more than 15 pages is extremely interesting, an editor may pass on it. Every journal has a limited number of pages available per issue. An editor cannot extend the page limits without incurring significant printing and mailing cost—extras usually not in her budget.

That means if an article is too long, someone else's article cannot be printed in the same issue. Only for an exceptional article will an editor decrease the total number of articles in an issue. Because any topic, no matter how well handled, is not likely to appeal to *all* of her readers, she is unlikely to bump other articles to run an extra-long article.

In estimating the length of an article, the author must consider tables and graphs. Because they take up more space than printed text, most editors only want to include the essential ones. As a rule of thumb, if the meaning of the table or graph can be given clearly in the text, there is no need for the illustration. A writer should use tables and graphs sparingly, only where they are essential to explain or clarify the data. Having said this, I am aware that there are a few journals with a preference for tables and graphs. If the writer is familiar with the journal where her article is going, she will know its habits.

An opposite space problem arises if an article is too short. Fewer than 10 pages may leave a gap in the pages devoted to articles. If an article is fewer than 10 pages long, the writer might think about formatting it for the "Letters" column instead. Conversely, a writer should not try to draw out a 3-page idea into 10 pages. Editors recognize padding.

APPEARANCE OF THE ARTICLE

In addition to providing clarity for an article, subtitles contribute to an attractive layout. If the article is long or complex, the writer should use subtitles liberally. Again, the journal guide will give the preferred style.

Another factor in appearance is the width of the margins. In this case the purpose is dual: wide margins give a good appearance as well as providing editors and reviewers with space for notes and suggestions. This goes for sides, top, and bottom as well.

The presence of corrections also detracts from an article's appearance. One or two minor corrections may be inserted in black print if necessary, though with computer-produced copies this can easily be avoided. Most computer programs will correct spelling errors. If one lacks a speller, the article should be read carefully for errors. Misspellings and typos are to be avoided.

These courtesies in manuscript preparation will not get a poor article published, but they will assure that an article is not dismissed before it has a proper reading. Taking the care involved in the mechanics of preparation is well worth the time. At the very least, the editor gets the impression that the writer is conversant with the rules of the game.

SUMMARY

The mechanics of preparing an article are important and can mark the difference between a good first impression and a bad one. Although the right format will not get a poor article published, it will avoid creating a predisposition to reject the article on the part of editors and reviewers. The writer who wants to be published will do well to avoid unnecessary mistakes that may decrease her odds in this era of stiff competition.

BIBLIOGRAPHY

Brosan, J., & Kovalesky, A. (1980, November). As the authors see it. *Nursing Outlook, 28,* 688–690.

Garrett, B., & Hawkes, W. G. (1992). Copyright—What's right? *Journal of Continuing Education in Nursing, 23,* 101–104.

Chapter 8

When Your Article
Reaches the Journal

A new author is often unsure what to expect once her article
has been submitted to an editor of a nursing journal. A little
knowledge of the process can save a lot of anxiety. No editor wants an author to feel that she has been left in the lurch. Any
time along the process, it is perfectly acceptable for the author to
call the editor concerning the status of her article. After all, the writer
owns the article; she has a right to know.

RECEIVING THE MANUSCRIPT

When a manuscript reaches a journal, it is usually logged into a
manual that tracks what happens to it from review, to evaluation,
to rejection, to acceptance or recommendations for revision, to
editing, to galleys or page proofs, to publication. Such a record
enables the editor to locate all manuscripts quickly.

The first correspondence with the writer involves sending an
acknowledgment that the manuscript has been received. Most but
not all editors send a postcard to this effect when the article is logged
in. The card will give no evaluation; it simply lets the author know
the article has reached the journal.

Then begins the long wait. Seldom will an author hear more until a judgment has been passed on the article, and that can take months if the journal is refereed.

IN-HOUSE REVIEW

For most journals, the first review is an in-house evaluation in which the editor (or assistant editor in the case of a large journal) reads the incoming article. In this reading the editor determines if the article has merit enough to be sent to the external reviewers. At this step the editor eliminates articles that are obviously not acceptable—such as those with extensive grammar/syntax errors, those with clearly outdated material, or material that is simply wrong.

In some cases, according to editorial policy, the editor will eliminate material that is unnecessarily inflammatory or hostile as well as material that is wrong for the format or style of the journal, for example, a research-type report sent to a journal not using this formalized approach. Additionally, some articles on overworked topics may be eliminated whatever their merit.

The degree to which an editor exercises discretion in the first cut will vary, but usually she will not send to the review panel articles that are obvious rejections. With few exceptions, professional journals use referees who volunteer their time to evaluate articles within their realms of expertise. These reviewers are well-known experts, subject to many time pressures. An editor is wise not to waste the panel's time with manuscripts having little likelihood of being accepted.

Once an editor has worked with her panel of referees, she gets a good sense for what articles will or will not be accepted. Indeed, she often has much to say about who is selected for the panel as well as the opportunity to orient them to the review function. The relationship between editor and panel is reciprocal, but not a relationship to be abused by passing on unnecessary work.

In the few cases where the editor is not a nurse and may feel unqualified to make the first cut, all manuscripts may be sent out to reviewers. This may also occur on a journal that is presently between editors.

If a writer receives a rejection quickly, it is likely that the manuscript failed to pass the first in-house review. The writer receiving such a rapid rejection probably needs to develop better writing skills or to select a different topic.

Although the writer might expect that an article with many flaws would receive an extensive critique, that is seldom the case. First-cut rejection letters often are brief, with terse comments such as "not for us." Few editors spend much time criticizing a manuscript with extensive flaws. In the case of a simple mismatch of article and journal style, the editor may, if she is so inclined, suggest more appropriate journals.

The degree of attention given to manuscripts receiving early rejection depends on the editor's time constraints and disposition. In today's market, every nursing editor reads many more articles than was the case in the past. Competition for journal space has become intense, and the paper flow over an editor's desk has increased 10-fold. Hence, she is likely to save her criticism for articles that have a better chance of resulting in publication. The author who receives a rejection with few comments cannot assume that the article had few flaws.

A word about motivation: All writers receive rejections now and then. The trick is to rise above them and keep on writing. The writer should learn what she can from each rejection and go on—either with the present article or the next one. Learning by one's rejections is just part of the process. If most nurses gave up the idea of being published after their first rejection, our literature would be slim indeed. Like falling off a horse, the answer is just to get back on. Write again; write fast.

THE REFEREED REVIEW

Most refereed journals have two professional groups that work closely with the editor. The first group, by whatever name, is the journal board, a group of experts who gives the editor general policy advice concerning the journal. Such advice may be offered in periodic group meetings or in one-on-one conversations between individual members and the editor.

The second group is the review panel. These are the professionals who read and rate articles. The review panel is usually comprised of a larger group of people than the journal board. Indeed, the panel may be extensive if the journal accepts manuscripts on diverse topics. In some few instances members of the journal board may also perform review functions, but most journals have two discrete groups.

Articles that pass the in-house review will be sent to selected members of the review panel, known also as the outside referees. This review process is much longer than the initial review. Usually a manuscript is sent to the three or four reviewers who are best qualified to judge its content. Before being sent out, all identifying information is removed from the manuscript. Hence, the reviewers are not biased by the author's name or credentials, or by the institutions involved if any. One of the joys in writing is that a truly good piece by an unknown author has an excellent chance of getting published. The blind review process makes this possible.

The length of time involved in the review process may be months, especially if the article arrives at the reviewer's office during school holidays (many are faculty members) or at a busy time, for example, the beginning or end of a school term. The busiest times for practice-oriented reviewers are less easy to predict, though summer vacations often bring slowed responses.

Most editors wait until they receive all reviews before making a final decision on an article, then consider the multiple responses together. Some editors use the reviews in an advisory manner, weighing heavily the specific comments made by the referees. Other editors simply count the votes to determine the fate of an article.

On clinical articles, the reviews are extremely important because an editor is seldom an expert in all the clinical arenas covered in received articles. One negative reaction might be enough to squelch an article if any clinical data are seriously questioned.

Often referees disagree on the value of an article and on whether or not it merits publication. In that case, the editor may suggest that the author rewrite the piece—to remove the bones of contention, to make it more orderly, to fill in obvious deficiencies, or to correct whatever flaws the reviewers have pointed out. A request that an article be rewritten, although not an acceptance, is a positive response. If the author in good conscience can make the suggested changes, there is a likely chance of publication.

If the suggested revisions are minimal, a second review of a revised article may be done in-house. If the revisions are extensive, another round of referees may be required. In either case, an editor is not going to suggest a revision unless she thinks the revised article has a good possibility of publication.

LONG WAIT

If many months pass between the postcard of acknowledgment and the correspondence of a decision, the author should feel free to call the editor. Sometimes the call will speed things along. Suppose, for example, that an editor does not look at an article a second time until all the reviews are received. Suppose one reviewer failed to receive the copy, and the secretary who handles the log fails to notice the delay in response. The editor, who has hundreds of articles on her mind, might not be aware of how much time has elapsed until the author calls.

Other accidents can happen. As an editor, I recall an instance when my journal moved from one location to another, and the moving company lost one box of articles and the log book. The blind reviews of these articles kept arriving, but I did not have the originals with the identifying information. I was forced to wait until the authors called to get the identifying information. One author of a good article took a full year before contacting me. A writer need not wait silently if too much time has elapsed.

GOOD REJECTIONS

If there is a positive side to rejections—and there is—consider that a slow rejection means the article passed the first cut and was sent to reviewers. Consequently, the writer may assume there was some merit to the piece, whatever its ultimate fate.

When sending a rejection, most editors try to give an author some idea of what was wrong with her article if time permits. The writer can use these comments for growth, either in relation to the present article or when composing subsequent ones. Many authors prefer to allow some time to elapse before working with these suggestions. After the disappointment has worn off, it is easier to handle comments with dispassion.

Editors handle rejection letters in different ways. Some send the author a summary of the opinions (theirs and the reviewers); others repeat the actual reviewer comments, even if they are scathing—or worse, inconsistent.

The author should think carefully about any suggestions from reviewers, but they are not to be taken as absolute dictates. A reviewer can make a mistake, be hesitant to try new approaches, or simply prefer a different style. Nonetheless, the author should give every suggestion careful consideration before dismissing it.

Reviewers and editors sincerely try to give an author clues as to what will make a piece publishable. That does not mean the author has to like what they say. Still, if an author desires to be published, she should seriously consider the merits of all suggestions.

Further, a writer needs to understand what "sells"—with reviewers as well as readers. I know, for example, of an author who wrote a very good article about why a nurse should be pleased and happy to play second string to a physician, including letting him be first author on articles she has written. The piece was well written, interesting, and made some good points. Yet in an era when nurses are trying to advance their discipline as a fully developed profession, it was predictable that the nurse reviewers would never accept it. This was not what the indignant author wanted to hear, but it was a fact in today's marketplace. Here was a case in which a nurse gored a sacred cow all right, but it simply was the wrong cow.

A writer also needs to understand that a perfectly good article may be declined even when it has few flaws, if it competes for limited page space with more exciting articles. Hence, an article might lose out to more interesting copy even though it lacked any definable flaws.

Unlike many editors, I always read every manuscript to the end, bitter or sweet (some editors stop if they are bored by the second page). But I have jokingly said—maybe not so joking at that—that if I have to force myself to keep reading, the article has little chance of success. Being accurate is not enough in today's competition; an article needs to be interesting too.

The subject matter also is important in a close decision. A good article on an overworked subject matter will often be sacrificed to give space to articles on more contemporary or unusual subjects. If the editor's comments lead an author to think that an article was a near miss, she may want to try another journal. First, however, she might consider ways to give the article a bit more spice.

Many first-time authors and some more experienced ones object to the fact that reviews are often critical in tone and content. If one searched, they argue, the critic could find something good to say about almost any piece of writing. Yet editors and referees seldom take the time to do this. Although it may disappoint an author, the lack of compensatory plaudits is the norm and probably a function of the time pressures faced by these busy people.

From an editor's perspective, it is more important to tell a writer what needs to be fixed than what works just fine. An auto mechanic takes the same approach. Nevertheless, it will be less frustrating if the writer expects criticism rather than praise beforehand. Even for the best of articles, an author is likely to hear only about the few details that need to be clarified.

TIMING FROM ACCEPTANCE TO PUBLICATION

Most editors try to make a reasonable match between available space and number of articles accepted for publication. Nevertheless, there are still some editors who accept more articles than they can publish in a timely manner. The duration between acceptance and publication may vary from journal to journal. On an average, the article in a nursing journal may be published anywhere from 6 months to upward of 2 years after its acceptance.

If a manuscript is held much longer than 2 years, it may become too dated to be used. When an accepted article is getting long in the tooth, an author has every right to negotiate over when it will be published. Some writers take back their articles if an unacceptable length of time is involved, and this is their right. Others reserve the right to update the article before publication. Sometimes the editor is the one to ask for an update.

The time between acceptance and publication may vary radically from one article to another even at the same journal. It is particularly difficult to predict the time lag with journals that use a different theme for each issue. In this approach, a journal tries to select articles centered around a single topic. Because many nursing journals are only published every other month or quarterly, a good article may have a long wait simply because it fails to fit the selected themes.

Other journals take a shotgun approach, preferring diversity in each issue. Even these journals seldom publish articles in the order of their acceptance. They will look for a balanced offering in each issue, that is, something for every reader.

By virtue of their subject matter, some articles demand fast publication, whereas others have more durability. I recall one sad case in which a good article on the American Medical Association's (AMA's) plan for registered care technicians had to be killed because the AMA rescinded this proposal just before the article went to press.

Sometimes the immediacy of the subject will ensure a fast publication. For example, an article that analyzes candidates' stands on health issues has to be published before an election. Most editors will give articles of this type an early publication date after an expedited review. (That means the editor calls on reviewers she can count on for a quick turnaround.)

Sometimes the fact that a journal uses a theme approach can work for an author. I recall a case in which a first-time author was published within 2 months of submission simply because her excellent article fleshed out the issue of the journal then under preparation. This author had the right theme at the right time, but she will surely be disappointed when next she submits an article and encounters the usual delays.

LEGALITIES

Once an article is accepted for publication, all authors will be sent releases to sign. Usually these releases do not commit the journal to publication but indicate intention to publish. As mentioned earlier, a topic—for example, a clinical procedure or a political stance—might become outdated prepublication, voiding the possibility of the article appearing in print.

The releases usually indicate that the author is giving the journal ownership or first publication rights, and that commitment should be taken seriously by the author. I knew of a case, for example, where an author falsified these releases. Her article was scheduled to be published on the same month in two different nursing journals. Rather than the enhanced publicity the author envisioned, she severely constrained her chances of ever being published again in the nursing field. Editors have long memories, and like other intraprofessional groups, they talk with each other. Nothing is more embarrassing to an editor than to find that an article held out as new by its author has already been published elsewhere.

Some authors think that if two articles contain some small differences in wording here or there, this is adequate to make each article an original. If the article has substantially the same content, an editor will not see it that way, especially because the publishing agreement usually requires the writer to affirm that the material is original and not previously published.

If an article has already been published elsewhere but an editor seeks to publish it again, the question of ownership arises. She must find out who owns the article—the original publisher or the author—and that depends on the agreement signed between them.

Permission must be acquired from the legal owner before a second publication is possible.

There are several instances in which a publisher might want to publish an article for the second time. Suppose, for example, an editor is preparing an issue on the theme of delegation. She might want to include an article on that topic that had become a classic. There are many instances in which an entire book is comprised of classic articles on a given topic.

Sometimes an article has been published earlier in a journal of another profession. For example, an article on nursing and the law might be republished in a nursing journal after it ran in a law journal. As well as obtaining permission, the second journal usually gives credit to the prior journal within the rerun article.

An author should consider carefully whether or not she wishes to sign away rights to her article. Most journals are content with first publication rights if the author prefers that arrangement. Although it sounds nice to own one's work, there is a downside to that decision. Some journals will not publish articles on a first-rights basis; they simply want to own everything they print.

And it is true that an article is more likely to be reprinted if a journal owns it than if a would-be publisher has to track down an individual writer. The journal has no obligation to update addresses of past authors.

An author does *not* own her article if it was a commissioned work. If a writer was paid to prepare and present a paper at a conference, for example, the paper belongs to that conference group. Often if a conference group does not publish the paper or sell tapes of the presentation, it may give the author permission to publish elsewhere. This requires negotiation in writing, preferably before the conference.

ERRORS

Another legal problem occurs when an article contains misinformation. In the worst sort of mistake, a dosage error, for example, the liability is dual; the author must not assume that responsibility passes only to the journal. Even if the dosage error occurred during typesetting at the journal, there is still author culpability. That is why it is particularly important that a writer read a galley proof with care.

Journals, especially those dealing with clinical matters, try to use great caution. Nonetheless, when an error happens and causes some harm, neither journal nor author is safe from prosecution. Neither author nor journal can be sued, however, for merely an erroneous printing. The printing must cause an actual error to be made in therapy, and it must be proved that the error caused injury.

EDITORIAL REFINING OF ACCEPTED ARTICLES

How much help will an author get from an editor once her article has been accepted? The answer varies, depending on the editor's time and inclination. Some journals have full-time editors, editorial assistants, and copy editors. At the other extreme, a journal editor may work part-time and do her own copy editing. Budgets vary as well as staff, and the amount of revising will vary accordingly.

Some editors are willing to take on an article with a good idea even if it is in poor form, though this was more likely to happen in past years when resources tended to be more plentiful. On the whole, most editors will not accept a manuscript that needs major revision unless the idea behind the piece is truly earth shaking. Often the only editing a piece receives will be a limited copy editing for grammar and syntax.

The degree of editing permitted by an editor's time commitments and budget will enter into her decision when it comes to accepting or rejecting an article that needs a lot of attention. Given this situation, a wise author makes sure her article is well written before submitting it.

Whether the editing is substantial or minimal, there will be rare instances when the author thinks her work has been changed in ways incompatible with the original intention. The author always has an opportunity to review, accept, or reject such edited changes.

Sometimes unacceptable changes are made by a copy editor unfamiliar with the buzz words in nursing. I recall a case in which a copy editor substituted *nursing practice* for *nursing process* everywhere the latter term occurred. The writer had been referring to a specific process, not to general practice as the copy writer assumed. The substitution was wrong and had to be changed back to the original wording.

The writer will learn of any proposed changes when receiving a copy-edited version of the article, a page proof, or a galley proof. The form received will depend on how the journal produces its issues and the cost of making changes at various stages of production. But every journal should, and for the most part does, afford the author the final word.

The author is responsible for carefully reviewing the suggested editing and approving or disapproving all suggested changes. Although a writer should not accept editing that distorts meaning, she should consider that the proposed alterations have been made by an editor or copy editor who streamlines articles for a living. Most authors appreciate the smooth flow that appears under a good copy editor's pen.

Still, any editor knows some authors who are oversensitive about alterations. A writer who is too fussy will probably have difficulty marketing her next article to the same editor. In essence, one is better off saving objections for places where they really matter.

Another sore point: Some authors grow indignant when they are given a short turnaround time for reading and correcting page proofs. (Sometimes a journal asks for a return the next day by express mail.) From the writer's perspective the journal has had her article for months or years. Why all the wait, then "hurry up" she wonders?

From the editor's perspective, however, things are different. Every day she is dealing with a massive amount of manuscript processing, all the while turning out finished issues of the journal, trying to keep within a tight publishing schedule. With few exceptions, publishing firms are no better staffed than are other businesses in this time of a tight economy. There will be enough staff to produce each issue—but just barely. And they will face the same sort of staffing stresses and delays that other people face. Burning the midnight oil around the time an issue goes to press is more the norm than the exception. And the writer will be expected to facilitate the process if at all possible.

Titles can be another source of difficulty. Journals usually feel free to change article titles, but the new version should not distort the subject matter. For example, a journal once changed a title from "sex crimes" to "rape," and the author was rightly indignant—her article was far more inclusive than rape. Yet on the whole, new titles are designed to enhance reader appeal. If a writer wants to keep her original title, she should make certain it is snappy.

Charts and tables also become bones of contention. Sometimes authors think charts essential when editors do not. Tables and figures take lots of printing space, and editors will usually eliminate them if the content is adequately explained in the discussion.

AFTER PUBLICATION

Sooner or later most accepted articles do get published, and the author has the reward of seeing her work in print. She should receive author copies (often two) of the journal or finished reprints of the article according to the journal's practices. Most journals provide opportunity for authors to purchase additional reprints at a minimal cost, though the author needs to inquire about this before the journal goes to print. Reprints made at the time of the press run are much less expensive than reprints requested later, requiring a separate printing.

Most professional nursing journals do not pay for articles, though some give discounts on future subscriptions or token payments. Usually seeing one's work in print is reward enough for an author.

Even better is the response an article evokes from colleagues.

If the writer receives interesting letters concerning the article, copies should be forwarded to the journal for possible inclusion in the "Letters" column. Some writers go so far as to ask colleagues to react to their article in print to make certain they hit the "Letters" column. Journals are always glad to receive thoughtful or interesting responses.

SUMMARY

The processes that occur between receipt and publication of an article are many and varied. It will be helpful if the author understands what is happening. Throughout this process, she has the right to be in contact with the editor and to know where her article stands in the processing. Most editors are pleased to keep an author informed.

The process of getting published can be a rewarding one if all parties know their rights and obligations. The editor–author relationship can be a positive experience if both parties understand each other's contribution.

BIBLIOGRAPHY

Gay, J. T., & Edgil, A. E. (1989, October). When your manuscript is rejected. *Nursing & Health Care, 10,* 459–461.

Smoyak, S. (1984). So what? . . . When editors criticize a manuscript. *Journal of PysychoSocial Nursing, 22,* 7–8.

Swanson, E. A., & McCloskey, J. C. (1982, fall). The manuscript review process of nursing journals, *Image, 14,* 72–80.

Part II

Writing the Book

Chapter 9

How Book Writing Differs From Article Writing

Most new authors start small, with articles, but some break the ground with a book instead. Even the writer who has completed several articles may feel like a novice when it comes to her first book. This chapter looks at the task of writing a professional book and how that differs from writing articles.

BOOK IDEA

In contrast to what happens with articles, almost no one determines to write a book, then casts her mind around for a subject matter. A book starts with an idea in the author's mind. Few would put forth the effort involved were it not for a commitment to an idea.

Often the idea for a book arises when the writer is unable to find a book that fits with her teaching plan or when she finds a dearth of literature about a clinical problem in her place of employment. When a nurse discovers that she holds some unique knowledge or is doing some aspect of care in a new and successful way, she may decide to communicate her expertise in a book. Dissertations often lead to books for this same reason: They involve something novel (see Chapter 11 for more about this). Or a publisher may request that a nurse well known for her expertise in an important area write a book on that topic. Commonly this occurs where the nurse has become a popular conference speaker or where she has published several well received articles on the topic.

Books normally deal with a larger corpus of ideas than articles. Some may be directed toward a single position like an article; many take a subject matter approach instead. Alas, some books deal with such limited themes that they would have been better presented as long articles.

Books with some sort of novelty have a much better chance of being published than the "me too" book that is just one more version on an old theme. Every book should have something special to offer to the reader; usually it is found in whatever gave the author the impetus to write in the first place. The nature of the novelty varies from book to book; it may lie in the content, the method of presentation, or in the accompanying teaching materials to name but a few possibilities.

KINDS OF BOOKS

Books come in many different kinds, usually but not always dictated by their subject matters. There are text books, books for practitioners, research reporting books, handbooks, manuals, workbooks, case studies, monographs, anthologies, and edited works of various sorts. Each form has its advantages and limitations.

Let us start with text books. Text books are written for students at various levels of nursing education. Often a writer's text is written out of the frustration of not finding just the right text on the market. Whatever their subject matter, each text is carefully designed to reach an audience at a specified level of knowledge of the content matter. Usually the text strives for a comprehensive view of its subject, while offering suggestions for further study. Bibliographies will be well developed, and footnotes are usual. Today's texts, except for nurses' aide and technician training, tend to use more references to research findings than was the case a decade ago.

In addition to pointing the way to other sources, a text often is designed with student learning activities in mind. For example, chapters may be introduced by formalized learning objectives, principles may be carefully explicated, and each chapter may close with a self-test or with a case study. One might think that text books were written for students, but actually they are written with faculty in mind. After all, it is the faculty, not the student, who selects the text. It would be interesting to know if the learning features that sell a book to a faculty member would have equal appeal to students making an independent selection.

Most texts are written for a particular course, and the text is likely to cover the entire scope of content perceived to constitute the course. The reason for that is simple: cost. A fundamentals text that only covers half the procedures taught to a beginning student, for example, would have to be supplemented with another book. Every faculty member knows that nursing students are not wealthy, and purchase of texts is a major budget matter. If one book will do, a faculty will seldom ask a student to buy two.

Some texts for advanced nurses can also be used by practitioners, but most books aimed at the practicing nurse are not texts. Books aimed at this audience lack the student learning aids; they are more likely to present "just the facts, avoiding cute learning devices. More often than not books for practicing nurses concentrate on a specialty too narrow to be suitable for a student audience. Or the book may have a particular slant or bias too controversial for a text. A book titled *Use of the Doppler in Modern Acute Care* would probably be too narrow for a student yet might attract nurses practicing in that specialty. *Curing Cancer Through Image Therapy* might attract nurses in holistic practice but could seldom be justified as a text in a course on cancer.

Just as nursing has developed *de facto* into specialized practice, so has the production of books for practicing nurses turned into a specialty game. The nurse in practice seldom buys a general book; instead she looks for books that will enhance her arena of practice. Moreover, she is likely to buy more specialty books than would a student. After all, she is earning a salary and establishing a career. Even though books for practitioners tend to be specialized, the specialty cannot be so narrow that the size of the potential audience precludes recouping the costs of production. More to the point, few companies will bother with an exceptional book if they do not think it will make a profit.

Research reporting books are another category. Each year some few books are produced based on a single research project or summarizing various research reports on a given subject matter. Research-based books are risks from the perception of the publisher because they tend to have a limited audience of nurses with a higher education. However, if the book focuses on an important subject, it may become a good seller. For example, the first volume of Waltz and Strickland's series of books, *Measurement of Nursing Outcomes*, was published by Springer just about the time when health care organizations were beginning to explore outcome phenomena. The subsequent volumes in this series continue to meet a ready audience.

Now and then a research book becomes an unexpected success. For example, Benner's *From Novice to Expert* had such dramatic implications for both education and practice that it became a major success for Addison-Wesley.

In addition to research books of this sort, there are texts that describe and teach the processes of research and metaresearch books that discuss topics concerned with research, such as how research has been used in the field, what research has been done in various decades, or new approaches to research. Some books discuss theory as it relates to other important subject matters, for example, theory and research or practice and research.

Research books are not all alike. Some, like the Waltz and Strickland series, focus on tools produced in research endeavors. A research book of this sort is invaluable to researchers or dissertation students seeking already constructed measurement tools. Other research books are compilations of research studies focused on results rather than tool construction. Some few books, like the Benner book, report a single research project.

Today many books on the market could be labeled handbooks. This category of book can be identified by its practical nature. Usually a handbook contains a consolidation of material or abbreviated subject matter too lengthy to keep in one's head. Carpenito's *Handbook of Nursing Diagnosis* published by Lippincott typifies the group, presenting a taxonomy of diagnoses with brief materials in each category.

Manuals are also practical, often presenting procedures and practices of a given institution. With the growth of case management, many institutions are producing manuals containing their case maps, for example. Other institutions have produced manuals with patient education materials, and some have even published nursing procedure manuals. Sometimes manuals are produced by publishing companies, but publication and sale by the organization creating the manual also occurs. Although many manuals on the market are produced by organizations, some are created by individuals. Like handbooks, manuals tend to have less run-on text than other books.

Workbooks are a form of book designed for extensive reader interaction with the materials. Some workbooks are designed to accompany given texts. A workbook gives tests, experiments, case studies, and other hands-on experiences for the user. Not all workbooks accompany texts. Some, like Fondiller's *The Writer's Workbook*, published by the National League for Nursing, gives run-on text followed by tests and exercises. Some workbooks leave plenty of empty space so that the purchaser can complete the exercises in the book itself; others do not. Some are published in traditional book form, whereas others are printed in loose leaf so that pages may be torn out. When using a workbook of this sort, one should be careful to honor the purchase agreement concerning whether or not such pages may be legitimately reproduced.

Books of case studies are popular, whether they stand on their own or serve as backup works for related texts. How much run-on text is included in a case study book depends on the author's preference. Some case books present various sections of content, each followed by one or more related cases. Others assume that completing the case study itself will convey content to be learned. Some books give right answers or discussions to be read after a case is completed; others do not. Some give no prior content and no discussion of the case but provide extensive bibliographies. Case study format is as varied as are the purposes served by these books.

Monographs are short books, maybe 150 pages or fewer; they are virtually extended essays, each published on a given subject matter. Often monographs are published by scholarly presses because their commercial value tends to be minimal. Costs in producing any book, whatever length, are high. Hence, these tiny books will appear to be priced high, given the amount of content. This fact turns off many potential purchasers. For this reason, it is not easy for an author to sell a monograph to most publishers. The new writer should not expect to get a monograph published unless it is a real earthshaker.

Anthologies are books that accumulate under one cover parts of works already published elsewhere (that is the most common source) in a collected volume dedicated to a given subject matter or theme. An anthology on nursing leadership, for example, might feature articles written by renowned nurse leaders that first appeared in journals. Not all anthologies focus on a content theme. One might, for example, find an anthology that publishes the most famous nursing articles of a given era or even an anthology that samples the work of a single author during different periods of her life.

The anthology entails a different sort of author commitment—a combination of selecting, writing, and the administrative details of getting a collection together. Like other books, it involves writing to some degree—the author must create the introductory materials—at least an explanation of why this material has been gathered together. Sometimes an author elects to write an introduction to each piece in the anthology; sometimes the function of each selection is assumed to be self-evident. In general, an anthology represents the editor's conception of the best available material on the subject.

The additional work on an anthology is both intellectual and administrative. First, one must know the subject matter intimately so as to make the right selections. Then one faces the nitty-gritty work of obtaining reprint permissions. Chapter 10 discusses the situation with anthologies and edited works in more detail.

An edited work is similar to an anthology in that it involves the work of several (or many) authors. However, the works may be written expressly for the edited book, or reprinted materials may be involved. Some edited works incorporate both new and reprinted materials. Sometimes it is difficult to differentiate between an anthology and an edited work; however, with an anthology the term *classics* usually comes to mind, whereas edited works tend to be more recent materials, not all of which is at the classics level. The label (anthology or edited work) is not as important as the fact that the editor knows what is intended with the work.

PROCESS OF WRITING

Not every author takes the same approach in writing a professional book. Some writers start at the beginning and write until the book is complete; others take months to organize a comprehensive outline before writing the first word. Still others write in bits and pieces tying things together and filling in gaps as the final tasks. All these tactics can be effective in the right hands.

We will focus in this chapter on the book produced by a single writer. However, the nurse considering producing an edited work or working with coauthors will find advice in Chapter 10.

Any approach to writing a book requires persistence. Books do not get written overnight, and few that are planned on a whim get finished. Completing a book requires a serious commitment of time and effort. In essence, writing a book requires sacrifice on the writer's part as well as on the part of her family.

A book may require persistence on the part of the author, but, in at least one aspect, it requires less workmanship than an article. An article must be terse and to the point. In a book there is room for digression and space for interesting side bars. One can be more wordy and get away with it. Yet the best books show where they are going; a book with a total lack of direction has little chance for publication.

BACKGROUND WORK

If the nurse has an idea for a book, she should go to a library and do a complete search for any other books that relate to her subject matter directly or even tangentially. With today's computerized search systems, most nurses can do a comprehensive search no matter where they live.

However she manages it, the nurse should read all the books that relate to her idea rather early in her own writing process. It is frustrating to discover later that someone had the idea first and has already written exactly the book one planned. Simply put, a book project is just too much work to redo something already done.

Conversely, some writers yield to a dangerous tendency: They follow other people's paths and tunnel their ideas into a book that looks exactly like all the books they have reviewed. They structure their table of contents around the same subjects, making certain they "cover" each item addressed by the other authors. This, of course, is the perfect formula for producing a "me too" book. That is why I think a writer should have at least an outline, a proposed table of contents, and a few finished chapters of her own before studying the works of others intensely.

MANUSCRIPT COMPONENTS

A book can be as unique or different as the writer dares to make it (provided she can sell it), but there is a traditional format that can be followed to give the book its structure. Its elements include front matter (title page, author's biography, dedication, table of contents, preface, foreword or introduction, and acknowledgments) the body of the book, and back matter (appendices, notes and bibliographies, and the index). We will look at these elements here.

Front Matter

Title Page

The work begins with a separate title page that bears the title and the author's name and degrees.

Author's Biography

Some books carry an additional one page biography about the author, sometimes titled "About the Author."

In the case of an edited work, the book may include a list of contributors. This list allows for a more extended biography than what appears in the table of contents, where just the authors' names and credentials usually appear.

Dedication

A writer should take advantage of a dedication page to recognize someone or some group near to her heart. Any publisher will gladly include a dedication page, but few will ask about it if the author does not think of it herself. A dedication is a good way to recognize those who helped with the book or suffered by the writer's lack of attention during its production. People can also be recognized in the preface, introduction, or acknowledgment sections that follow.

Table of Contents

A table of contents is an important component in the book. A well-organized easy-to-follow table of contents can make the difference between a reader deciding to buy a book or putting it down in disinterest. (It has the same affect on potential publishers, book reviewers, and award judges too.) The table of contents cites by page number and title all of the subsequent sections of the book, including all parts and chapters. If the book is an edited work with numerous authors, it is common to list the author's name and credential after the appropriate chapter(s).

Except in a large tome, possibly one with a thousand or more pages, it is not common to give pages for smaller sections than chapters. Nevertheless, some large textbooks may give page numbers for sections of chapters. A medical-surgical text, for example, might give pages for subordinate disease conditions or nursing diagnoses appearing in the respective chapters, themselves divided according to major body systems (book parts).

In scholarly works, the table of contents may be followed by a list of tables. Or a work that is heavily illustrated may list photographs, artwork, and other illustrations.

Preface, Foreword, or Introduction

Often today, the terms preface, foreword, and introduction are used interchangeably. But there are important distinctions.

The preface or foreword both serve an orientation function. However, the preface is by the author of the book, and a foreword is by someone else—usually some expert whose recommendation (it is hoped) will improve book sales. It may give the reader some personal insight into the author, telling, for example, her background, why she wrote the book, or any significant aspects of work involved in producing the book that are not in the body of the work. Often acknowledgments to those important in the creation or production of the book are included in the preface. Such acknowledgments may be limited or extensive, depending on the circumstances.

All books should have a preface. And a foreword is good to have when the right conditions permit. The author must be sensitive to the circumstances when asking an expert to write a foreword. First, the author must provide the expert with a full copy of the manuscript. One should never expect a recommendation to be based on friendship alone. In most cases, an expert will not be asked to write a foreword unless she has personal ties with the author. However, there have been cases in which editors have intervened, using their influence to find an expert willing to do the job. In seeking a foreword from an expert, the writer must be sensitive to issues of competition. If the writer's book will be in competition with the expert's own books, it is better not to ask this person to write the foreword but to find another expert.

If the book has been produced under the auspices of some group or committee, the foreword may be written by an authority from that group. This provides the author with an opportunity to recognize the support given to the book and provides the organization with a deserved voice. It also orients the reader to how the work came to be.

In later editions of a book, it is common practice to repeat the prefaces from the earlier editions, with the order working backward from the new preface. At times, this practice is scrapped, and only the preface to the new edition is given.

The term *introduction* may be used to cover the same content labeled preface elsewhere, but often an introduction relates more directly to the text to follow. An introduction orients the reader to the body of the text. If the introduction is lengthy, it may be titled, "Introduction," but presented as the first chapter. If short in length, it may simply be labeled "Introduction," with different content in the first chapter.

Acknowledgments

Sometimes a writer chooses to have a separate, single page for acknowledgments. These differ from the dedication in that the person or persons recognized in the dedication may not have been directly involved in production of the book. Acknowledgments are extended to those who were instrumental in creating or producing the book.

One might, therefore, find a dedication to the writer's parents and an acknowledgment to her secretary/typist, for example. (We already mentioned that acknowledgments could be included in the preface if the author prefers that format.) Both elements (dedication and acknowledgments) are optional.

Body of the Book

The body or text of a book contains the essential content or subject matter. In a small book, the body may be given a simple format, that is, divided into chapters. In a more complex book, there may be several parts, each containing chapters.

Where parts are used to organize the chapters, each part may begin with a written introduction, or the part may simply be given a title that is assumed to be self-evident. In this case, there may be no explanation on the page in the text that presents the title of the part. In either case, a new part gets a separate page from the preceding or following chapters.

Most books today use a system of including references and bibliographies within the text, most commonly at the end of each chapter. In nursing, the format of the American Psychological Association (APA) (APA, 1983; Gelfand, 1990) seems to be the most commonly used one, but there are still companies that use other formats. The author who does not know who will eventually publish her book is probably safe with APA format. For a small book that has few if any references, all references and the bibliography may be given at the end of the total text instead of chapter by chapter.

The body of each book will be unique, depending on its contents, and the writer should not feel bound to follow any particular convention. The objective is to present the book in the format that makes the most sense for the reader.

Back Matter

Appendices

Appendices, if any, follow the body of the book. This is the place for tangential materials or extended reference materials that are too long or complex to include in the text. Often appendices include forms or extended charts. Appendices are usually but not always materials that might be used in connection with several chapters rather than just one. In nursing, appendices often include care plans, quality measurement tools, grading systems, and the like.

Notes and Bibliographies

When there are few notes and limited bibliographies, they may be placed together in the back matter instead of at the end of each chapter. More often, they provide additional sources relevant to the subject of the book. These may be important sources that did not link directly to quotes or comments in the chapters. Bibliographies in this section may simply give titles of books and articles, organize these sources according to topics or chapters, or even give annotations concerning contents.

Index

The index gives all the page numbers where any major subject matter or author appears in the book. These citations may be organized separately by subject and author or combined into a single list. An index is optional, although it can be invaluable to students and researchers. Most textbooks, scholary books, and books for professionals have one.

The writer may provide her own index topics or rely on the publisher to create them. Most companies will provide indices, charging the author for the service off the top of her first royalty payment.

If a writer has never constructed an index, she is probably better off to let the publisher do this task. People who index books for a living simply do it better, certainly quicker, than a new writer. The writer will always have the opportunity to go over the index for additions and to correct errors.

FINAL PRODUCT

A word about the final product: A submitted book manuscript is expected to be complete down to the last comma. True, a good editor may suggest revisions and copy-editing changes, but the manuscript reaching the publisher should be as close to a final product as the author can make it.

Magical Thinking

Some writers exercise magical thinking about a book manuscript—submitting it with missing or incomplete references or sections marked with notes like, "I will finish this section closer to the time of publication so it will be right up to the minute." Trust me, there is no magic fairy at the publishing house who will run to the library to find the missing citations nor one who will nudge the author to supply the missing pieces "now." The editor will simply bounce the copy back to the writer for completion. Most houses will not touch a manuscript until every chapter, every section, has been completed. One simply cannot begin a complicated processes like editing and publishing without a complete manuscript.

Format

A final manuscript, carefully paginated, is submitted loose in a box not much bigger than the manuscript itself. In this day of desktop printing, some authors think an editor will be impressed with a copy done like a book, possibly bound and using fancy fonts, italics, all the bells and whistles. This is difficult to work with, however, and is the last thing an editor wants.

Use the simplest, clearest available font, and double-space with wide margins. Underline rather than italicize. The editor will recognize this as a professional job.

SUMMARY

Producing a book is a major event in one's life. The writer will be living, breathing, digesting the book for well over a year in most cases. One should not underestimate the drain on oneself, one's family, and one's social life—let alone one's career.

From the idea, through the research, drafting, revision, and negotiation, writing a book is an exciting venture. Whether one uses traditional forms or breaks new ground, producing a book is an investment that is usually well repaid when one receives the first copy hot off the press.

REFERENCES

American Psychological Association. (1983). *Publication manual of the American Psychological Association* (3rd ed.). Washington, DC: Author.

Gelfand, H. (1990). *Mastering APA style: Instructor's resource guide.* Washington, DC: American Psychological Association.

Chapter 10

The Edited or Coauthored Book

There are at least three basic author arrangements for books. The simplest is that in which a single author writes a manuscript. Chapter 9 was written from this perspective.

The second type of book is coauthored, with two or more contributors. Usually these authors work together producing a single manuscript that is attributed to all the authors but in which individual efforts are not distinguished for the reader.

A small deviation in the principle of author anonymity may be seen in the prefaces of these books, where each author may add her comments under her own name. In a well-written book of this sort, the reader should not be able to tell where one author leaves off and another begins. Where the writers have served as respective editors for each other's contributions, the work often becomes seamless.

The writing team is a common phenomenon in nursing, and many excellent books have been produced in this fashion. The most common form of the coauthored book is one where two authors work together from the start.

On other occasions, the original author or authors discover that their expertise is inadequate (sometimes a good editor helps them draw this conclusion), and they take on additional authors to supply the needed knowledge.

It is difficult for more than two or three people to work on a manuscript together in this format, simply because it takes so much coordination. Nevertheless, there are several well-known, coauthored nursing books written by threesomes. More common by far is the coauthored book with two authors.

A special form of the coauthored book is one in which the first and original author is not interested in turning out a new edition of a book and takes on a second author for purposes of providing the updated edition. This may also occur when an original author of a classic book is deceased.

If the first author is still involved in the newer edition, there is a need for a precise agreement concerning who will do what and how royalties will be divided. Where the newer author is responsible for all additions and updating (probably the most typical arrangement), royalties are often split on a 50-50 basis. Many factors may enter into such negotiations, including how much of the original book requires updating.

The edited book is a different form of joint effort. In this format, the individual contributions are credited to their respective authors, with one or more persons serving as editor(s). Editors take responsibility for selecting the topics and authors, preparing the book prospectus, organizing the book, writing prefaces and other front matter, and generally tying the pieces together in a coherent manner.

Edited works may involve new contributions on the part of all writers, or they may collect already published materials selected to fit under a single subject matter. Some edited books combine these two sources, using some new and some reprinted materials. Editors may or may not add their own chapters to the collection.

EDITED BOOKS

Many a new writer has calculated that an edited book will give her a relatively painless publication in a short period. These writers are usually disappointed. The truth is that every form of book has its own rewards and difficulties.

Edited works require great perspicacity in selecting contents, then careful structuring so that the chapters fit together as a unified whole. Often this effort consumes as much time as writing one's own ideas alone. Indeed, I know of one prolific writer who claims her most difficult book was one that brought together already published classics on a given subject matter. She ended up having to glean 20 articles from about 500, carefully considering the balance and the need for comprehensiveness in the collected work under production.

Works of Prepublished Materials

Editing a work that uses already published materials requires much more "bookwork"—tracking down who holds copyrights on every piece used, obtaining permissions, and the like. Often an edited work contains materials that first appeared as articles in various journals. Commonly, journals hold the copyright on pieces they have published, but that is not an absolute rule. Increasingly, authors are extending the right of first publication rather than copyright to journals.

In those cases, the editor will have to locate the author of the article, who half the time has moved, died, or cannot be located. (In this section, when we speak of the "editor," we will mean the author/editor of a collected work, not the editor assigned later by the publishing house.)

When a journal owns the copyright, there is usually a fee for reprinting an article as a book chapter, possibly a few hundred dollars (though this fee has been increasing lately). The editor must expect to invest some "up-front" money in obtaining these permissions.

Even where a journal holds the copyright, it is common courtesy to inform an author when her article has been selected for inclusion in an edited work. Not every one remembers this formality, however. I can think of several times when I have found chapters of my work appearing somewhere unexpectedly.

In one incident, I was merely browsing through a book, happened on a chapter and read three pages (thinking how much sense this author made) until the material began to sound all too familiar. Ready to be indignant at plagiarism, I turned to find the author's name only to find it was myself—a piece for which a journal held the copyright.

Some authors forgive the editor who includes but does not tell. Nevertheless, there are some authors very interested in seeing how influential their work becomes, and its adoption in edited works may be of great interest to them. Indeed, for faculty members pursuing promotions and tenure such reprinting may add clout to their portfolios for advancement.

New Contributions

When an author/editor solicits new contributions instead of publishing already printed works, she finds herself dealing with a different set of problems. No matter how carefully she has thought out the selection of authors, some of the writers are sure to disappoint her.

First, not all of those the editor selects as contributors will agree to provide a chapter. Sometimes a would-be contributor simply does not wish to be associated with the particular editor. For example, a well-known nurse author may prefer not to be included in a book published under the name of an "unknown." In a kinder vein, the best-known nurse writers simply get more requests for chapters than they can possibly honor.

Another factor that vexes some would-be contributors is the usual royalty distribution policy. Most book companies prefer to give authors of individual chapters a one-time payment. Often that payment is token to say the least—a few hundred dollars, typically. Payments are kept modest for good reasons, say the book companies: What if the book does not sell? No publishing company wants a heavy up-front investment. Thereafter royalties are distributed only to editors, and, if the book sells well, they may be substantial.

From the publisher's perspective, this system makes sense: It is simple and deals with only one or two people. After all, no publisher wants to have to figure out percentages and send out 20 royalty checks to 20 different authors every six months for as long as a single book sells.

The contributor, however, may see things differently. She may see an author/editor getting rich on her hard effort. (It is always the case, that whatever one's role in a book, one's own part seems the most difficult, the most deserving of recompense. And I say that as someone who has been both book editor and contributor over the years.)

Furthermore, the editor must expect that some would-be contributors will fail to keep writing commitments and deadlines. (Remember, the motivation may not be high, given the recompense.) One fail-safe system is to notify all contributors in advance of the action to be taken in that contingency. Setting irrevocable time frames is one way to handle these human frailties. Clear-cut deadlines may be given to each author with an understanding that, if the assigned date is missed, the writing will be handed over to someone else. Needless to say, if one makes a single exception to this rule, the system fails.

Let us suppose the would-be editor gets over the bumps involved in acquiring the desired authors for her book. Now she faces an even more difficult problem. She must deal with her authors' diverse personalities and egos (the latter come in various sizes). Worse, character and contributions intermix, and a young editor may have great difficulty in rejecting an inferior chapter dashed off hurriedly by a famous nurse. Quality control and person control demand infinite patience and tact.

One way to handle the quality control effort is to set up a system in advance in which submitted chapters are reviewed by a small panel. This is one way to reject an inferior chapter while diffusing the resentment of its writer. This approach only works, however, when the authors know the rules from the start.

Let us imagine the best scenario: The editor has successfully rejected the unacceptable chapters and found good substitute authors. Now comes the editing. Few book editors are willing to take even a good chapter "as is." Some chapters may be good in themselves but miss the mark—namely, they may veer from the special focus envisioned by the editor. Now the editor is in the position of asking a busy author to redo a major piece of work.

Needless to say, the new writer who tackles the editorship of a book will soon learn that the work involved is more than the mere collection of chapters from willing colleagues. Putting together an edited book can be a humbling lesson in the politics of human relationships.

Collected works always land the editor in the middle, requiring a special sort of tact and intellectual honesty so that a common purpose surmounts interpersonal frailties. A delicate balance is required to keep all authors happy and feeling that they have been treated fairly at the same time. To achieve this while preserving the quality of the work almost requires a genius. The effort involved is seldom less work than the effort required in writing a book alone. The difference is simply a matter of which sort of problems one prefers.

COAUTHORED BOOKS

Most coauthors form great working teams, making the best of their collegial relationship. Because these joint efforts work, there is little need to discuss them. Teams who do not work well together usually strangle each other early in the production process, precluding creation of the proposed book. But it is a sad fact that futile would-be coauthorships have ended a lot of valuable friendships. Often it is the friend one most values with whom it turns out to be impossible to work.

Coauthorship seems to be like marriage: wonderful or awful. Because it is impossible to tell which way the arrangement will go, I suggest—like a premarital contract—a prebook contract, written or verbal, but clear. Decide ahead who owns the book idea, who has the right to go ahead, possibly with another coauthor, if this relationship fails. Decide ahead how or if the second party will be recompensed for the time and effort put into the book before the split.

Get an agreement fostering honesty—namely, that each party will freely voice resentments when they form, and that each party will have the right to call it quits without having it affect the friendship. Sometimes the best coauthor is an acquaintance instead of a friend. With an acquaintance, it is easier to hold relations to the business of producing the book.

In addition to getting some sense of equity concerning who will do what, one also needs an agreement concerning whose name will be first and whose second. Do not wait until near publication for this decision. Do not try those artificial sops—drawing names from a hat or using alphabetical order. Usually partners are not exactly equal, and they have to make the difficult decision of who is most deserving of the top spot on the marquee. Is it the one doing the most work? The one having the original idea? Make the decision in advance. If the accountability and effort involved shift, the decision may need to be discussed again. See chapter 14 for some of the problems involved in ranking authors.

NEED FOR A UNIFIED STYLE

Chapter 14 also reviews the need for a unified style in every book. Somehow even in the edited book, where different authors contribute different chapters, the book must feel like a single work, not a motley collection. Where chapters are being written especially for the book, sometimes unity is be achieved by setting a similar structure for each chapter. For example, some books start each chapter with objectives and end with a practice exercise; others have the authors apply the same internal categories to discussion of different subjects.

Uniformity also may be attained by having each writer take the same slant on the subject matter: not coronary care, for example, but coronary care *made easy*. This sort of approach, if carried out by every author, will give a sense of homogeneity to the manuscript.

Other books achieve that sense of uniformity because the editors build linkages between chapters by introductions. Sometimes the editor writes an introduction for each chapter, sometimes for parts under which related chapters are gathered. These sorts of linkages are critical in the book that relies on reprinted articles that cannot be modified.

A cogent introduction can explain why these five articles have been selected—for example, what principles their inclusion illustrates, how they complete each other, or even how they offer different perspectives on the same subject matter. What matters is that the reader know why these readings appear here.

Uniformity of style is important in a coauthored book too. If you can tell which member of a team wrote which chapters, then the integration is not complete. Figuring out who wrote what is a game publishing house editors play frequently, incidentally. Not that one aims for homogeneity as the only overriding principle. But the components of the book must fit together so that the reader comes away with a sense of completion, with a feeling that the book has delivered on its topic.

SUMMARY

The edited or coauthored book presents special challenges. Although the writing task is distributed among two or more authors, the collaborating and communicating tasks increase 10-fold. The advantage of having a convenient peer review must be balanced against the danger of human frailties surfacing on all sides.

Perhaps the best advice to the writer it to "know thyself." A writer will soon learn which sort of book will give her more satisfaction: a joint endeavor or a solitary work. The naive reader or even the new writer may assume that edited and coauthored books "split" the effort. In fact, they may come closer to doubling it. For writers who like the action and stimulation of being involved with lots of other people, however, the coauthored or edited book may be the answer.

Chapter 11

It's a Great Dissertation, but Is It a Book?

Just as some writers think a term paper is an article, some writers think a dissertation is a book. Often these nurses with new shiny doctorates have been encouraged by dissertation chairmen to seek publication. Indeed, many have been assured by well intentioned faculty that their dissertations merit publication.

Whether or not the work merits publication, it will almost never be publishable in its original dissertation form. Every year, hundreds of authors simply bundle up copies of their dissertation and send them out to publishers. With only a rare exception, these authors are due for a disappointment.

Even in those rare cases in which the content of a dissertation is of paradigm-shaking importance, the formats for dissertations and books are unique, serving different purposes. Only if a publisher is absolutely enthralled with an idea behind a dissertation will she request that the material be rewritten in book format. The writer has a better chance of succeeding if that work is already done and the dissertation has been converted to book format before it reaches the publisher.

DIFFERENCES

What are some of the simple differences between books and dissertations? There are many, ranging from purpose to presentation to style. We will look at the main ones here.

Purpose

A dissertation is written to prove that the author is capable of designing and executing at least one research project, applying at least one research method. The topic of the dissertation is secondary, important only to the extent that it demonstrates that the author knows how to select a researchable topic and can carve out an appropriate research question within the topic.

Books, conversely, are about their subject matters. Frankly, no one who buys a book is interested in judging a fledgling researcher's capacities. That is why faculty are paid workers instead of volunteers. Indeed, when a purchaser buys a book based on a research study, she *assumes* that the research is valid and will be angry if she detects flaws in the methods used or conclusions drawn. The research must be right, but that is only the beginning.

Books sell on the basis of ideas, not on the research skills of the writer. People buy books to learn something new, not to examine the writer's prowess.

Scope

Of necessity a dissertation deals with a limited topic; otherwise the author has not yet adequately narrowed her topic of inquiry. There is a touch of truth in the old quip that PhDs know more and more about less and less.

It is true that any dissertation, appropriately refined, will have a small audience of interested readers. These will be other academics with specific, limited interests in the narrow research topic. Because of their backgrounds, these people will have the skills to get the dissertation from the rather extensive retrieval systems now available whether or not it ever gets published.

A book, conversely, must appeal to a wide audience of readers. Otherwise it simply will not pay to produce it. Usually this means that the book cuts a wide swath, has a wide scope. This is not to say that all dissertations fail to have universal interest. But it is the rare topic that captures a wide readership. Sometimes a narrow study has wide applications or implications that make it sell. Whatever the reason, if a dissertation does not have wide appeal it will not convert into a book.

It does no good for the author to rationalize that hers is a subject that every nurse *ought* to know. People do not buy books that someone else thinks they should own; they buy books that answer their perceived needs or desires.

Format

Although certain scholarly journals publish research articles written according to the research method, even they cater to a limited audience. Such a format is a sure loser when applied to a book. Let us face it, dissertations are designed to be boring.

First of all, dissertations are repetitive. We are going to hear about sample size, for example, when methods are discussed. Then we are bound to hear about it again under demographics. And it will be mentioned again when the author discusses implications—she will be careful to consider her sample in saying how far and to what general populations her findings can be extended. And that is only one element: sampling. A dissertation is a fine interweave of elements—back and forth repeatedly.

Books, conversely, try to make each statement only once. They are dynamic and flow forward, not back and forth. Repetition is boring; a boring book doesn't sell.

Also, let us face it, there is something about the research format that brings out the pomposity in the best of us. Just try to be humorous and chatty in your dissertation and see what your chair says! Academe is such a serious business, or so it must appear.

Carts and Horses

There is an even greater flaw in the research format than built-in boredom. That has to do with the order in which things get addressed. For most of a dissertation the reader is up in the air. A problem has been presented, and darned if we know when or if it will ever be solved.

Even when an academic reads a dissertation, does she plow through all that data collection before finding out the answer? Not a chance. As soon as she finds the research question, she turns to the last chapter to see how it all came out. Only if the answer interests her does she go back and check on the accuracy with which it was produced.

In other words, a dissertation starts with a horse (a research question) and works toward the cart (the answer). But a good book, other than those you buy through the mystery club, goes in the opposite direction. The amazing conclusion is what sells a book. Books put carts before horses.

Conclusions

Speaking of conclusions, few dissertations come up with earth-shaking findings. Often what they prove is what common sense told us all along. It may be good to have proof that our common sense was on target, but, frankly, that will not sell books.

Yes, a dissertation that disproves its exciting question is just as good as one that does not. That is what research is about. But it is not what book sales are about.

If the topic *and* the findings do not clear channels for new ways of doing or seeing important things, the dissertation simply will not sell as a book. Yes, it will serve a valuable niche sitting there among the other entries in dissertation abstracts, but it will not be made into a book.

CONVERSION PROCESS

Okay, suppose one has a great dissertation; how does it get converted into a book? Ninety percent of a book that centers around a dissertation is going to deal with the findings and implications, particularly the implications. The gut work of the dissertation, the part the student labored over for months or years, will probably be summarized in a puny chapter. That goes for the literature review, too. Essential citations will be worked into the text, but most of the literature review will end up in the bibliography.

A reader asks, how does this information affect my practice? Implications and applications; that is the game. Unfortunately, because the dissertation process is taxing, the student is likely to run out of steam just when she reaches the implications section.

Faculty, alas, are more willing than they ought to be to allow this flaw to pass. But then faculty are human, already bored with this dissertation, and acutely aware of the new bunch of recruits knocking at their doors. Nursing empathy enters the picture too—Suzy has been working on this dissertation so long, and she really wants to graduate before she gives birth to those twins. Okay, we will forgive the faculty.

In essence a book starts with the findings and implications, gives a quick review of the study methodology, then goes back to its main business: more analysis of the implications and applications. Its final goal should be to show nurses a way to do their jobs better or provide new information rather than to show how well the author performs research.

To be interesting, a writer may have to go beyond the strict implications drawn in her dissertation. Indeed, some of the best books to come from dissertations do not even mention the fact. If the idea of the dissertation was bold, the writer may get further simply exploring all the ramifications without being bound by the limitations of the original study.

This is not to say that a research base *cannot* be a source of strength for a book. Look, for example, at Benner's successful research-based book, *From Novice to Expert* (1984). But it sold not *only* because of its research base (which was excellent) but because of its far-reaching implications for the practice of nursing.

BOOKS ARE TO SELL

As chapter 12 explains, books are business more than pleasure—at least when you are trying to get a publisher interested. Unfortunately, the quality of the research in a dissertation and the work's prospects for selling may have nothing to do with each other.

Well-intentioned faculty do not always know that much about publishing, so they tend to encourage students to publish based on a dissertation's quality. In a better world, all worthy dissertations would be published, but we are not there yet.

Furthermore, there is nothing wrong with being represented in the library as an original dissertation. The writer's work will still be read and appreciated by those most in a position to appreciate it. No royalties, alas, but it is an imperfect world.

Finally, an author does not need to give up simply because a dissertation is not right for book format. Most dissertations can be adapted to article format. Some dissertations actually serve as the source for more than one article. Chapter 15 looks more closely at writing from research.

SUMMARY

Dissertations can be converted into books, but doing so is not much less work than writing any other book. Yet if a dissertation is to have a chance at publication, the conversion must be completed before it reaches the publisher's desk.

Further, not every dissertation, no matter how good, is likely to be published as a book. To qualify it must be of practical use to enough nurses to make publishing it economically worthwhile.

REFERENCES

Benner, P. (1984). *From novice to expert: Excellence and power in clinical nursing practice.* Menlo Park, CA: Addison-Wesley.

BIBLIOGRAPHY

Binger, J. L., & Jensen, L. M. (1980). *Lippincott's guide to nursing literature: A handbook for students, writers and researchers.* Philadelphia: J. B. Lippincott.

Blancett, S. S. (1986). Getting your research published. *Journal of Nursing Administration, 16,* 4.

Chapter 12

Producing the Book Prospectus

This chapter looks at the nitty-gritty of producing a book prospectus, the marketing document designed to sell the proposed book to a potential publisher. The prospectus is really an essential first step. Too many disillusioned authors have gone ahead and written an entire book—a major commitment of time and effort—only to find out later that no publisher was interested. Marketing a prospectus prevents this sad outcome.

Many of the decisions involved in organizing the book prospectus are essential decisions that must be made for a successful book anyway. Creating a prospectus is not really extra work as much as making important decisions early in the writing process. The prospectus becomes the underpinning, not only for selling and marketing the book but also for planning it.

A good book prospectus can make the difference between a sale and a rejection. The prospectus typically ranges from 25 to 75 pages depending on the nature of the book. It is the main document used by publishers in deciding whether or not to purchase a book. Indeed, most prefer to receive a prospectus rather than a completed manuscript. Even when a publisher agrees to read a manuscript, the writer may be asked to prepare a prospectus because it addresses many aspects beyond the mere content of the work. Many publishers have their own guide for creating a prospectus. An author can get a copy with a simple request.

Although an idea is a great place to start a book, it is important to find out early whether that idea has any chance for publication. It is not uncommon for an author to submit a manuscript only to find that the likely publishers already have books on the topic under production and are not interested. Or she may discover that publishers are uninterested because they think the book has little likelihood of being profitable. A prospectus can prevent this sort of frustration.

The writer should prepare the prospectus as soon as she knows how she will compose the book. Indeed, the prospectus may help shape the book by clarifying her intentions, finalizing her structure, and firming up the book content.

Unlike an article, a book prospectus can be sent simultaneously to many publishers. It is important, however, to see that appropriate publishers are selected. A quick review of past publications by a company will tell an author whether or not her book fits in a publisher's line. Appendix B lists some of the major publishers of nursing books.

The author can request book catalogs from the selected publishing houses if access is not available through other channels. Often librarians have these catalogs. Publishing house catalogs enhance a computerized library search. The latter only list present holdings; company catalogs list upcoming books as well.

The writer will need to get to know every published book that even tangentially relates to her proposed book. Recent and upcoming publications as well as classics that are likely to compete should be identified. The author needs this information for the prospectus as well as for selecting potential publishers. The knowledge gives her clues as to which houses publish books in the general area where her book fits; it also reveals which publishers presently lack a book on her specific subject matter.

Once an author has decided which publishers to query, she is ready to request their guidelines for writing a prospectus. The following discussion describes the areas usually included, but the author should follow the publisher's preferences.

CONTENT OF THE PROSPECTUS

A prospectus starts with a working title, the author's name and credentials, then a concise description of the project, namely, a few paragraphs conveying the idea of the book and a few more explaining why the author is the best person to write it. Relevant aspects of one's career and education should be identified here. Ideally, the introduction should be given on one page, providing a quick summary sheet. The editor, who may see hundreds of manuscripts within a short period, will appreciate having this at-hand summary.

The introductory page is separate from the letter that conveys the manuscript. Some authors omit such a letter, assuming that a submitted prospectus speaks for itself. An introductory letter, where used, is brief, identifies the author, the working title of the book, and asks whether or not the editor might be interested in publishing the work.

Some authors are afraid to put their ideas for a book in writing lest they be stolen. Although no one can say it has not happened, editors of established firms are honorable. They have a sincere respect for the written word and are sensitive to ownership issues.

Table of Contents

After the introductory page, the next section in a book prospectus (order may vary from publisher to publisher) is the annotated table of contents. Here each chapter is titled and followed by a paragraph or two describing its content. The description should give precise details, not generalities. For example, one would not say that a chapter will discuss common nursing theories used in ambulatory care. Instead, it would identify the specific theories to be discussed.

If the book has multiple writers, the author for each chapter should be identified. For an edited book, all contributors should have indicated in advance their willingness to write the assigned chapters. A prospectus does not merely list authorities the editor hopes will agree to write once the proposal is accepted.

A writer must give serious consideration to the organization and sequencing of her book. Many a book proposal is turned down because the table of contents lacks coherence. No publisher wants to work with a disorganized writer.

The table of contents shows any obvious flaws in the book's conceptualization. An editor not only looks at the content proposed for each topic but also considers the topics as a whole. Are they comprehensive enough to cover the subject matter? Are there any glaring omissions? Is there any chapter that does not seem to fit? Are the chapters offered in an order that makes sense?

Special features

Either within the annotation for each chapter, or separate (before or after the table of contents), the author should describe any special attractions or teaching/learning strategies used in the book. For example, if each chapter starts with objectives and ends with review questions, that should be identified. If each chapter is to be shaped by the same format, it is acceptable to describe the format once instead of repeating it for every chapter. If the features vary, then it will be necessary to identify them individually in each chapter annotation.

At present new publishing arrangements are being created for computerized books (with continual updates sent out on disk), books used in conjunction with computer assisted instruction, and books that interface with all sorts of audiovisual components. Others texts are devised with tests that must be mailed to a central source for grading, or, more traditionally, books that are meant to be used in conjunction with one or more workbooks.

Although such special features may be important to the author, they may limit the number of interested publishers. Many mainstream publishers are not interested in such complex products. Conversely, a book company owned by a corporation that also makes audiovisual products might express interest in some of these unusual formats.

Elements, such as photographs, graphs, tables, cartoons, or illustrations, should be noted in the special features section. These items add to the cost of production but they may also, when used effectively, add to the book's sales potential.

Any feature other than run-on text should be described under special features. If photographs or illustrations of a unique kind are to be used, samples should be included. Photocopies will do in most cases. The writer should never include the only copy or only good copy of a photograph or illustration in a prospectus.

In the case of illustrations, the author needs to ask whether the publisher will provide them. In the prospectus, she may submit amateur drawings that can be passed on to an illustrator. If the company does not supply artwork, they will have artist services to recommend to the writer. However the artwork is arranged, amateur work is not acceptable in the final copy. If any service is expected of the publisher, this should be identified here.

Sample Chapters

No matter how clever the book idea or how much a book may be needed, no publisher will acquire a book if the author is not competent to produce the required content in effective language. Good sample chapters may not get an author a contract, but poor ones will definitely lead to rejection.

The writer is usually expected to supply two or three completed chapters. These chapters allow the editor to see the quality of work of which the author is capable.

Some writers pick the first three chapters for submission; others pick what they consider the three most critical chapters. Most editors will be more interested in the quality of the writing than in where the chapters occur in the book.

Multiple Authors

If there are two or more authors, then one or two chapters by each author should be included in the sample chapters. The only time this will not apply is when each chapter is to be written by a different contributor. Books of the latter sort may be difficult to sell unless the contributors are well known leaders in the field. Books proposals for such contributed works should be sent with some writing samples by the editor, especially if she is both editing and contributing chapters.

As indicated in chapter 10, books with multiple authors are managed several ways. Sometimes the work is presented in its entirety with no identification of who wrote what (a coauthored book). In other cases, a separate author is identified for each chapter (an edited work).

Curriculum Vitae

Curriculum vitae should be included for all authors, editors, and contributors to a proposed book. They should be written so as to make clear each author's special experiences or preparation for writing the given chapters/components. Prior publication credits should be included as well as credentials, present and past affiliations, and applicable work or life experiences.

Marketing Factors

This section of the prospectus identifies and characterizes groups likely to purchase the book. It is to the author's advantage to identify as many sales targets as possible while still being realistic. For example, if a proposed book is slotted for nurses with a particular kind or level of nursing expertise, this should be made clear. If it is intended as a text for a given level of education, this also should be specified.

Editors are cautious when an author makes grandiose claims that her book can be used for every level of nursing student from freshman to doctoral candidate. They are equally skeptical about an assertion that the same book can serve specialists and generalists. Such a book may exist, but it is a rarity. An overblown assessment of the book's sales potential is unlikely to convince an editor. And it will not give the publisher a clear idea of the book's market.

Some authors make the opposite mistake of considering their work from too narrow a perspective. A graduate-level text on coronary care nursing, for example, might have features that make it adaptable for continuing education courses. The writer should be creative but realistic in thinking of potential readers. One useful tactic is to divide the market analysis into primary and secondary targets.

Competition

Sometimes an analysis of competing books is discussed under the topic of marketing. Wherever its placement, this analysis is an essential part of a prospectus. In this section the author analyzes her book's place in relation to books already on the market. In what ways is the book different from its competitors? In what ways is it better? How is it going to stand out? What unique aspects will help the sales force? What will make nurses, faculty members, or others select this book instead of its competitors?

It does little good to say that the book will be better, newer, longer, or shorter than the competition. These are conclusions, not explanations. The author must describe the differences, allowing the publisher to draw his or her own conclusions. The usual format for this section of the prospectus is to analyze the most popular competing books, telling their advantages and limitations and how the proposed book differs from them.

Obviously the author must have intimate knowledge of the competing books to do this effectively. Few publishers will be interested in a "me too" book with few unique aspects. We all know that numerous books get written on the same subject matter; however, in each case, some author has had to convince a publisher that her book was unique enough to carve out a sizable portion of the market. Finding out the selling points of competing books is a necessary part of composing a book prospectus. The author has to carve a separate niche for her own product.

In writing this section of the prospectus, some writers play down the competition and praise their anticipated work excessively. One should keep in mind that the editor knows the field well and is unlikely to be impressed by this tactic. A realistic critique of how a book stacks up with the competition will impress an editor with the author's knowledge of the field.

If a book happens to be the only one on the subject matter, this should be emphasized. Even then, the writer should identify the most similar books—even if they are different from the proposed one. If one's book is truly one of a kind, the odds in favor of publication rise—provided the topic is likely to appeal to a wide audience. It is an editor's dream, seldom realized, to produce a book with no competition and a large reading audience.

Formatting

This section of the prospectus presents the size, shape, and printing requirements of the book. Length is the most important question, and pages may be estimated in either printed page or manuscript page. Manuscript page estimates (double-spaced, regular printing font) are more accurate because the correlation of manuscript to printed page varies based on size of the printed page and type size used by the printer.

Because most manuscripts are typed or laser printed on 8½- × 11-inch paper, page estimates are fairly consistent. One should not use elite (small) typeface. If an editor asks for word count instead of a page count, figure about 250 words per manuscript page of run-on text. The size of a completed book manuscript typically ranges from 250 printer-generated or typed pages upward to thousands. If a manuscript is under 200 pages, one may be looking at a monograph or slim edition.

It is more difficult to sell books at either extreme of the spectrum. Excessively large tomes bear a high price tag and involve a major publishing effort. Such books, usually clinical, have a greater chance of being published if they are written by known authorities in the field. Other than clinical texts, it is difficult to find a market for such weighty books in nursing subjects.

A small book presents a publishing problem for another reason. One must ask, will the target audience be likely to invest in a small work? Certain fixed production costs do not go down in direct proportion to book size, so they must be calculated into the purchase price. Small books cost the purchaser more per printed page, and this may mean a price that inhibits sales.

For this reason, many publishing companies issue few small books or monographs. Academic presses may publish significant, ground-breaking monographs or small books as a service to their constituencies, even if the works are unlikely to turn a profit.

Most important, the size of a book must be right given its subject matter. Although purchasers will pay a substantial price for a large clinical text, they are less likely to do so for a book on nursing's public image, its history, or nursing theories. Whether one approves of buyer choices has little to do with sales, and a publisher acts on the facts, not on what an author thinks purchasers ought to do.

Determining the size of a book is usually a publisher's decision, but in certain workbooks or books with unique artwork size may be dictated by contents. Authors of workbooks, for example, often want a book with large pages and lots of empty space for making notes.

Scheduling

At least two dates should be given in the scheduling plan of the prospectus: the date when the first draft will be completed and the date when the author expects to deliver the final manuscript to the publisher. First-time book authors are notorious for underestimating these scheduled deadlines. One cannot just estimate the time needed to produce the three sample chapters and multiply by the number of intended book chapters. Inevitably, this seemingly logical method fails. The initial chapters tend to be written in a mood of excitement and high interest that is difficult to sustain over the long haul. Structural problems, research difficulties, lagging interest, fatigue, and intrusions from the author's life inevitably intervene and slow down the production pace.

The time when the final manuscript is delivered will be less important for some books than others. Some technologies and care dictates change rapidly, and a book that reaches the editor a year later than promised may be rejected for outmoded content.

As in other aspects of the prospectus, the scheduling should aim for what is realistic. And no editor has ever complained if a book arrived on her desk ahead of schedule. For the average book, a new writer will do well to set herself a 1-year deadline for completion. That time frame will sound reasonable to a publisher, and it gives the writer a clear target for which to shoot.

Most but not all editors want to see a completed first draft. After reading it, an editor can give the writer a good idea of whether the book shows signs of living up to its promise. At this stage an editor can suggest corrections for problems the writer may have failed to detect.

Authors who have written books before, especially those who have worked with the same editor on prior works, may elect to skip this step of the procedure, submitting only the finished manuscript.

SUMMARY

A good prospectus is the first step in getting a book published. As much thought must go into preparing the prospectus as into completing the book. Not only does the prospectus give the author a product to sell to the publisher, but it provides a road map for completing the book.

Often a first-time book writer fails to appreciate all the work that will be involved in writing a book. A good prospectus forces the author to come to terms with many of the decisions points. The effort put into preparing a good prospectus pays off in the final product and may spell the difference between getting a publisher or being rejected.

BIBLIOGRAPHY

Bly, R. W. (1991, July). The bulletproof book proposal. *Writer's Digest*, 33–37.

Chapter 13

Finding and Working With a Publisher

Now that we have looked at writing the book and the prospectus, we will assume that the author was fortunate and attracted several publishers. Next it is time to consider both the selection and how to make the best working relationship with the publisher and the book editor. While we are at it, we will take an overview on the whole process of producing a book.

BENEFITS OF BOOK WRITING

The effort involved in producing a salable book has at least two major payoffs lacking with articles. First, there is the likelihood of making a serious contribution to one's profession—not that a hallmark article cannot do the same. However, it is far more likely that a book will have significant impact simply because it can say more.

Second, there is the prospect of financial compensation—a benefit seldom achieved in writing professional nursing articles. Book royalties tend to range anywhere from 7% to 17% although a new writer is not often in a position to negotiate the higher figures.

Compensation, incidentally, is only loosely connected to the book's inherent worth. Instead, remuneration is directly linked to the number of sales. Hence, a rather ordinary book teaching fundamentals of nursing may garner higher royalties than an exquisite book designed to educate nurse executives. The numbers are easy to calculate: There simply are more students (more potential purchasers) than there are nurse executives.

Few nurses write strictly for a profit motive. For most authors, a cost-benefit analysis would indicate an enormous amount of work for a comparatively small direct financial payoff (royalties). For faculty members, there is a secondary financial gain in those cases in which book publication leads to promotions and increments in salary compensation.

Whether they work in education or practice, most nurses who write professional books get great personal satisfaction from the effort, and, yes, some enjoy the prestige and status that tends to come with book authorship.

FINDING THE RIGHT PUBLISHER

The truth is that most first-time book authors do not so much select a publisher as fall in with one. If only one publisher expresses interest in the book, the selection makes itself.

There are two choice points in picking a publisher. The first involves deciding where to send a prospectus, the second (if one is fortunate) selecting among interested publishers. For our purposes, we will treat this as a single decision point because one should not send out a prospectus to a company without first having decided it would be a satisfactory publisher for one's book.

In a sense the book prospectus is the counterpart of the query letter, with some important differences. Analyzing a book prospectus is a major time investment for a book publisher. Unlike the query letter, a writer should not use a shotgun approach of sending out large numbers of copies. It is acceptable, however, to send out copies to more than one publisher if each publisher is informed in the cover letter of the number of other publishers who have received copies for consideration.

Limited multiple submissions, with acknowledgment of the fact, is acceptable. Most publishing companies, incidentally, will not be interested in reading a prospectus if they know it went out to many publishers. Again, it is a question of how each company chooses to invest its limited human resources.

Like journal editors, book publishers and editors talk to each other. The author who thinks she can send out 20 copies of the prospectus to 20 different publishers that will never know the difference is mistaken. Indeed, such tactics may defeat the purpose. Honesty is the only policy.

Hence, a writer will send out two or three copies of the prospectus at best, and they will be sent to houses that the author would be happy to see publish her book. Appendix B lists some publishers that handle nursing books.

Let us assume that the writer is ready to submit her prospectus. How does she make a selection of publishers? The first approach is that age-old one of asking friends who have already been published. Were they happy with the editing services, advertising, and royalty arrangements of this company or that one? Do not expect, however, to find an author who thought the company did enough advertising for her book—from an author's perspective, there is never enough advertising.

In asking various authors about their publishers one gets the vital writer's viewpoint. This may be an easier task for a faculty member than for nurses in the practice arena simply because faculty tend to be surrounded by other writers. If she does not travel in circles that provide easy access to other authors, a nurse can ask prospective publishers to put her in touch with some of their authors. Of course, there is a Catch-22 here: Most book publishers will not extend this courtesy until they are already interested in a prospectus.

There is nothing to stop an assertive nurse from contacting authors on her own if she has a means to find their addresses. Usually letters sent to an author in care of her publisher will be forwarded. Whether an author so contacted will respond is anyone's guess.

Let us assume the writer relies on a publisher to provide the introductions. Even though the publishers will select authors they think were most pleased with their services, the writer will still get a sense of the differences among houses if she talks to enough authors from each.

She should remember to ask not just about personal treatment and editing services, but also about marketing efforts, attention to book design, and pricing strategies employed. She can also ask about prospects for paperback versus hardcover copies.

If she talks to enough authors, the writer begins to see that publishing companies are not all alike. Some houses baby an author through the whole book production process, whereas others are more like an assembly line. Sounds like a simple choice, does it not? Who would not prefer to be pampered? At least until one discovers that the "assembly-line" publisher may be willing to produce twice as many copies of the book. And that a third company will give the book a bigger advertising budget.

And so it goes. The right publisher for one author is not the right publisher for another. One author will be greatly concerned for the quality of the product in terms of design, cover materials, and size. Another author will not even want to be involved in such decisions—just produce lots of copies, sell them, and keep those royalties coming. One author will rely heavily on her editor; another will rage if he suggests too many changes.

Talking to nurse authors is only one source of input. If the nurse has the opportunity to visit publishers' booths at a convention or book fair, her task will be made easier. At each publisher's booth, she can browse through a wide selection of books. And she should not miss any of the handouts. Picking up numerous book companies' publication catalogs provides a quick way to compare and to discover the unique interests of each house.

The writer should not merely browse and pick up literature, however; she also should talk to the book company representatives tending the booth. She can ask questions about the books in the same category as her projected work. She might ask which of their books in this category are best sellers. And would they be interested in another book on this subject?

Some businesses send employees low placed on the organization chart to represent them at conventions. That does not happen to be true in the book industry. The new author is likely to find major book editors, heads of marketing, and even some publishers themselves at the booths.

The writer should use this personal exchange opportunity not only to find out about books already on the market but those under production and scheduled to come out in the near future. More important, she can respond to the personalities, their interest—or lack of it—for her project. She can get a good idea of which companies impress her as potential publishers for her work.

Variables That Affect Choices

Whether talking to authors or company representatives, there are several factors that dominate an author's conversation and her subsequent choice. First she will want to consider the royalty percentage offered by each publisher. As stated earlier, most royalties range from about 7% to 17%, but a new author should not expect an offer at the high end of the range.

Even if financial gain is her chief objective, the nurse cannot be guided by royalty percentage alone. A house that provides good marketing support may sell more copies of her book, making up for a lower royalty percentage point. Pricing of the book may also affect her profit, and errors can be made on both sides: a book priced too low to earn much or a book priced too high to compete with other books on the same subject.

Nor is finance the whole question. Different publishers treat their authors differently. Some have a mass-production mentality in which the author will get little beyond a cursory copy editing.

Other houses give exceptional service, assigning an editor who provides manuscript advice and editing, working closely with the author to produce the best book possible. If professional recognition and prestige are primary objectives of the writer, such full service might help the author win special attention in the forms of awards or exceptional reviews. Such an author might, for example, review the *American Journal of Nursing* awards for the last few years. How many awards has the house she is considering taken?

Picking a publisher involves weighing a lot of incommensurate factors. Even with concerted investigation, the new author probably will not get a full sense of what all those factors are. The only realistic advice that can be given is to get as much input as possible, then dive in.

Author Beware

There are some warnings that can be given to a new book writer. First, there are a limited number of publishers who specialize in nursing books. If a nurse goes through her library (home or school), she will quickly become familiar with the common publishers' names (see Appendix B). Firms that publish lots of nursing books usually have been successful at it.

At any given time, there are a few companies moving into the nursing field or marginal companies trying to hold onto a slim nursing collection. These book companies will be actively searching for authors and, for that reason, may do a better job of wooing the prospective writer than does an established house.

The author may need to weigh this special attention against the hard facts of company experience—not to mention the efficiency of their distribution channels. Is nursing a sideline for the company, an endeavor that will not get much of its marketing budget?

This does not mean it is always a mistake to go with a publisher who's a "new kid on the block," but the author needs a clear idea in advance of the support the company is able provide in production and distribution. Unfortunately, a new writer may have little basis on which to make a judgment. Conversely, if the only offer she has is from a "start-up" firm, she may have little to lose.

Given any other alternative, it is bad business to contract for a nursing manuscript with a house that has never before published any nursing books. Nor should a nurse assume that a publisher that has previously handled related health care fields can automatically handle nursing books effectively. For example, a publisher that has previously only marketed medical texts to physicians has little or no "edge" in starting up a nursing line.

Conversely, if one were writing a health-related book for the general public, one would not select a house that only publishes nursing texts. Again, the advertising and distribution channels would be wrong. Nursing publishers are long on marketing lists of nurses but usually short on marketing lists of general consumers and inexperienced in marketing to this target audience.

Finding Out Who Publishes What in Nursing

Whatever sort of book she writes, the author should seek out a publisher who produces books in more or less the same category. Some publishers do not want books too similar to those already out under their signature. These publishers prefer not to put their products in competition with each other. A house that produces one of the leading texts on staff education, for example, might not want another book on that subject. Yet they might be delighted to consider a related text on computerizing routine staff education programs.

Other houses do not see internal competition as a problem. They are comfortable or even eager publishing several books in the same category to develop strength in this area and attract first-rate authors.

Whatever she finds to be its editorial position on this issue, the nurse can be guided by the general type of books that a house publishes. For example, she would not send a clinical book to a house that only publishes nursing management and leadership books.

YOU ARE IN BUSINESS

One difference between articles and books is that book writing immediately puts the author into the business end of publication. Unlike an article, a book is something that costs a publisher serious up-front investment. And publishing houses are not in business to lose money.

Every book accepted for publication involves two assessments on the part of the publisher: the assessment of the quality of the book and the assessment of its value as a marketable product. Will it earn money? How much?

Every publisher knows how many copies of a book they must sell to break even or to make a profit. That cold fact will influence publication decisions. Nor is the break even/profit point the same for every publisher; many factors from production processes to advertising policies affect it.

Some publishers have the luxury now and then of publishing a book for which they predict a financial loss. They only do this for a landmark publication they feel is so vital to the nursing community that it should be published despite poor financial projections. Other publishers—most of them—will not or cannot commit to a projected financial loss.

PRODUCTION PROCESS

The production process has many components: the contract, delivery of the manuscript, work with an editor, marketing, and distribution. The following discussion will touch on each of these elements.

Contract

Work on a book begins with the signing of a contract between writer and publisher. Often a contract is offered on the basis of a prospectus and a few sample chapters. A new writer may wish to discuss the contract with a lawyer or with other authors who have signed contracts in the past. In truth, most book publishers use standard contracts that vary little from one to another. But the writer should have the contract reviewed by someone knowledgeable.

Few professional writers use literary agents, but where an

agent is employed he negotiates the contract. The chief reason that few agents are used in publishing books for professionals (as opposed to the lay public) is that, unlike a writer of fiction, a nurse author can get her book read without an intermediary. Further, an agent's fee cuts into an author's profits—and nursing is not a field where an agent is likely to get a better deal than could the author alone.

Most publishers are willing to negotiate if any particular contract item presents a problem for the author. They may be more willing to make changes for the well-known author than for the newcomer.

Copyright

An important contract issue concerns who will hold the copyright for the book, the author or the publisher. The publisher will usually file this document unless an author makes a point of reserving this right for herself. Some publishers will even file in the author's name if requested to do so. Who holds the copyright matters little except in the rare case of an ownership dispute, for the publisher's rights are established in the book contract, not by virtue of the copyright.

For authors wishing to file their own copyright, forms can be obtained from the Registrar of Copyrights, Library of Congress, Washington DC 20559-6000. The cost of filing until January of 1996 is $20. Some writers feel more secure holding their own copyright, seeing it as protection against theft of the work. In truth, I cannot remember a single case of such a theft of a professional book in my career.

Usually what new writers actually fear is the theft of a clever idea, and, fortunately or unfortunately, ideas cannot be protected by copyright. One safety factor is that a person who would steal an "idea" is seldom willing to do the hard work of writing the book to go with it. Sometimes authors *think* their ideas have been stolen when, in fact, the same idea occurred to someone else at the same time. Almost every editor has a tale about a time when she received a prospectus on an arcane subject matter, only to receive two more on the same subject matter within weeks.

Delivery of the Manuscript

If the writer lives up to her part of the contract, her work will be published. That includes finishing the book in the agreed-on time frame with the quality of writing and organization demonstrated in the prospectus. One could argue that a writer would be foolhardy to proceed with a book without the assurance provided by such a contract. Nevertheless, a book contract is far from a firm deal.

If the quality of the delivered manuscript does not live up to the promise of the prospectus, the publisher has reason to back out of the deal. And the publisher will be the one to make the judgments concerning whether or not the book has lived up to its promise.

Another contract breaker is an author's failure to produce the book on time. If the book is submitted a year later than promised, the publisher may not have allotted production funds for it in the present budget, or, worse, the book editors may have decided that the subject matter is no longer timely. Either way, it is up to the publisher to decide whether or not to accept a book that failed to arrive on the projected date.

Writing a book is a serious project involving much more work than writing even a long series of articles. First-time book authors have been known to underestimate the time involved by as much as a year or more. Many nursing books are "in the works" for two or more years. Excessive delay on the part of an author, of course, risks making the book obsolete before it is even published.

Another risk in being late is that one's idea may first reach the market in the form of someone else's book on the same subject matter. Competition is a fact of life in writing books, and the first book out on a new topic has a distinct advantage. If the writer's delay has allowed a competitor to get out a book on the same subject, one's publisher may be a lot less interested in publishing the book than was the case when the contracts were signed. Being late with one's commitment under these circumstances might be fatal.

Some authors think they can meet a promised deadline by submitting a partial manuscript. "Here it is, I just have to add that chapter on legislation and that tiny section on how to negotiate with the nurses' unions. I'll get that stuff to you within the month."

These words are not music to an editor's ear. Even if a partial manuscript is received, it will be set aside until the completed work is received. And do not expect your editor to insert and paginate late-arriving materials either. The best policy is not to send anything until you can send everything.

One word of caution concerning when a manuscript arrives: Often an editor sets a delivery date based on a notion of how timing affects sales. For example, a book that arrives a month later than anticipated may be too late to be on the market in time for September classes (a major sales time for texts). For a fundamentals text that may mean virtually a year's worth or royalties foregone. For other books, cycles in the industry may not matter.

Timing can also relate to a book's subject matter. Some books are designed to optimize on a popular trend of the moment. Past trends might have included such once "hot" items as assertiveness, empowerment, restructuring, or reengineering to name only a few trends that approached fadlike proportions. If a book is designed to cash in on a fad, it must reach the publisher fast. If the fad dies before the book reaches the publisher, it will never see the light of day.

Working With Editors

We will assume everything goes well, and the book is delivered as promised. Next the author begins a critical association with her editor. With luck, the author will work with a single editor throughout the production of her book. The editor is the writer's contact point thereafter. The editor's involvement may differ from house to house. In some publishing firms the editors do everything, right down to copy editing. In other houses, the editor simply oversees the book production, calling on other experts (possibly even subcontractors) at various stages of the process.

For a book, we can loosely identify two different sorts of editing. The first is macroscopic and done by the book's editor. In this editing, the work will be read for content, sequence, and missing or misplaced themes. This editor reads from a comprehensive view of how the book will and should look in its final version. Major revisions may be suggested at this time.

Later, after the book is in its final version, the author will receive copy editing on a sentence by sentence level. Copy editing has more to do with the grammar and syntax than with the ideas and organization. At times it is difficult to draw the line between these two levels of editing. This is particularly true in those instances where both functions are done by the same editor. Such separate treatment also may be minimized if a book arrives in such good condition that the editor does not think it needs anything but copy editing.

One of the best or most irritating relationships for the author can be with the copy editor. Most copy editors are exceptionally skilled at their work, but every now and then an author–copy editor rift sets in. When this happens, the best solution is for the writer to ask for a change of copy editors. (I am assuming here that the writer is not simply a prima donna.)

Sometimes a new author is like a woman with a first baby: She thinks her production is perfect in every way. This may make for disillusionment when she receives back the edited copy of her manuscript for approval. The answer is usually to learn to take a good dose of humility—without letting oneself be pushed around.

To understand the copy editor's suggestions, the writer will have to learn the common proofreader's marks and what they mean. These are available in many places, including the *Publication Manual of the American Psychological Association* (3rd ed.) (1983). The writer might as well own this or Gelfand's *Mastering APA Style: Instructor's Resource Guide* (1990) anyway, as most nursing books follow this style manual.

Proof Reading

The book author will likely see two copies of her work in progress. The first set will be her originals with editing suggestions added.

This is an important set because it provides her only chance to compare the original with the proposed changes. An author has the right to reject any proposed change, but usually she will find the editor's suggestions enhance the book.

The next copy will be galleys or page proofs—in other words copy set in print as it will appear in the bound book. These pages arrive all at once or in pieces, depending on the editor's predilection and production schedule.

Page proofs must be read with exceptional care. Sometimes an author is so thrilled to see her work finally "in print" that she is less than thorough in reading the proofs. Remember that the accidental omission of a word like "not" can change the writer's whole meaning. Read carefully!

Another word of warning: By this time the author, if the truth be told, is rather sick of her book. She has read it more times than she would like to remember. It is easy, therefore, for her to see on the printed page what she wrote rather than what is actually there. Take a sentence like this: "When applying a nursing theory to patient care, the staff nurse should should be careful to pick a theory that compatible with her value system." For the reader, the two errors stand out (one word repeated and one word omitted), but to the author who knows this sentence by heart, it will be more difficult to see the mistakes. As she reads, she tends to automatically make the corrections, literally not seeing the errors. Experienced writers know this hazard; new writers need to be warned to read carefully.

Timeliness counts in proofreading too. The author will usually have a short turnaround time in which to return the edited materials. If she is going to be out of town for a week or on sabbatical in Helsinki, she should make sure the editor knows where and how she can be reached.

Marketing

A word about marketing. Somewhere near the end of the production process, the author will receive a questionnaire from the marketing department. Some writers fill out this document in a cursory fashion. Do not! The document has a direct effect on how a book will be marketed and how well it will sell. Thoughtful consideration must be given in answering all questions if an author wants a successful book.

In addition to working closely with the marketing department, a writer can do much to advance the sales of her own book. For example, if she is presenting a speech or workshop on the book's topic, she can make certain that copies are available for the audience to purchase. Or she may arrange a book autographing party at her home or place of employment. Or she may request that friends send reviews of the book to likely journals.

Some authors promote sales by using their books as the text in courses they teach. If a book has been written with a given course in mind, that tactic makes sense. Personally, I prefer to use someone else's text as the main required book in a course, simply because my lectures may be based on my book content. I think this gives the students a more balanced view: mine and someone else's.

Distribution

The last step in the book process is distribution. The author cannot do much about a company's distribution channels, but she can inquire about the process. If she sees any major flaws, she is free to make suggestions. At least she will have given the company an idea of where the book should be distributed if she filled out the marketing survey with care.

Sometimes a writer has access to mailing lists that the company lacks. It never hurts to compare. Or she may know of major conferences where her book might be displayed and sold. An enterprising author can increase sales with a little creativity.

There is one other distribution before the royalties start rolling in (usually in twice-yearly payments, no tax withheld); that is when the writer receives her author's copies in the number specified in the contract. There are never enough copies of the book, so the writer should be careful how many she promises to friends. (I have been guilty myself of giving them all away—though I only made that mistake once.) Usually the contract includes a clause enabling the author to purchase additional copies of her book at a reduced rate.

With luck, the author receives her author's free copies before the book goes on sale, though things can go wrong. I remember being surprised to find one of my books on sale before I received copies. I soon got over being miffed, however. What author can object to her book being sold?

SUMMARY

Getting the right publisher and editor will make the book production flow a lot more easily. There is no magic formula for finding just the right fit, but the writer can approach the search in a systematic and informed manner.

Further, she can understand that production of a book is a two-way street in which both publisher and author have rights and obligations. Every author needs to know the steps involved between the writing of the manuscript and its appearance on the bookshelves of her local stores.

REFERENCES

American Psychological Association (1983). *Publication Manual of the American Psychological Association* (3rd ed.). Washington, DC: Author.

Gelfand, H. (1990). *Mastering APA Style: Instructor's Resource Guide.* Washington, DC: American Psychological Association.

Part III

Special Issues

Chapter 14

Writing With Colleagues

Many nurses get their first taste of writing for publication when they get involved in a group activity resulting in a publication. Writing with others is not a bad way to start, provided one has a good understanding of the rules of the game and the possible pitfalls. If it is well planned, collegial writing has much to offer the new nurse writer.

WHY MULTIPLE AUTHORSHIP?

Writing efforts that involve two or more authors occur for many reasons. Sometimes an inexperienced writer seeks a more experienced partner because she feels the need for a writing apprenticeship. Sometimes this happens when a nurse has a good idea but is insecure concerning how to communicate it. In this pattern, the inexperienced writer (the content expert) negotiates with a writing expert.

If the content expert is not a good writer, in most instances it is not necessary for her to take on a coauthor merely to refine or make her work publishable. There are numerous people, nurses among them, who make their living as editors, helping writers who feel the necessity for this sort of assistance. Use of a hired editor is certainly preferable to giving someone else shared credit for one's ideas. Remember, an article or book is simply a vehicle to carry ideas; it is the ideas that really matter.

Most nurses are capable of putting their ideas into words without the aid of an editor. Professional journals do not expect the level of writing expertise one sees in published fiction. Professional journals expect clear language that sets forth the message in terms and in a sequence the reader can understand.

Yet all decisions about authorship are matters of degree. And there may be instances in which an editor does more than simply refine someone else's words. If the editor helps the author shape and refine her ideas and explore their implications, it may be that shared authorship is warranted.

Other collegial writing efforts may emerge as a final stage in a shared project, perhaps a program design or a research project in which several people participated. The writing may be seen as only one component in a coordinated set of activities. The writing may be assigned to one or more of the project participants even though all names will be included as authors. Shared authorship recognizes that participation in the other aspects of the project has importance at least equal to the writing/reporting component. We will discuss the rules for determining such importance later.

There are cases in which a student who is writing a publication based on a thesis or dissertation may feel her committee chairman deserves to be included as a coauthor in payment for services rendered during the study. We will return to protocols for this later also.

The point is, in all collegial writing it is necessary to differentiate between authors and actual writers. Ideally, authorship should be reserved for the owners/possessors of the knowledge conveyed.

WRITING ABOUT A NEW IDEA: WHO HAS RIGHTS?

On any project, care must be taken not to misrepresent ownership. Sometimes a young writer, failing to understand the subtleties of ownership, hears about a project underway and publishes information about it before the project participants are prepared to do so.

For example, the well-known author of a popular self-help book was sued and required to turn over the profits from her book to the researcher who had shared his findings with her, never suspecting that she would publish them in the popular press before his more scholarly work on the subject was completed.

My personal experience included a similar event. I was chagrined to find that about 80% of a book written by one of my students was based on lecture notes from my classes. Somehow the student had failed to understand that plagiarism involves stealing ideas as well as specific words.

Indeed, I had been using the classes to test the content for my own book on this particular subject. Needless to say, I was astonished to find my notes, almost verbatim, released under the student's name. Although I decided against it, a lawsuit would have been an appropriate response.

WHO SHOULD BE AN AUTHOR?

Not all participants in a project qualify as authors. Take, for example, a project where patients received different teaching programs concerning their hypertension. Suppose there was a nurse whose assignment was to meet with patients, orient them to the project, and assign them to the different counselors who administered the various teaching protocols. The nurse might even have collected the demographic data on the clients. If she were not involved in design of the project, creation of the teaching programs, or interpretation of the data collected, however, her role was incidental despite her heavy involvement.

One way to reward participants who fail to qualify as authors is to acknowledge them in the article. Editors will be pleased to insert an acknowledgment that describes the contribution of such persons. As a matter of fact, an editor will prefer this strategy to publishing a list of authors so long as to be awkward.

WHO GOES FIRST?

In authorship, the sequence of the names is almost as big an issue as who will be included. There is no easy way to determine ranking. There is no doubt that the sequence of names makes an important statement to the outside world. In many promotions hearings, for example, more weight will be given to the first author than to second and subsequent authors.

Furthermore, some journals, frustrated by long lists of innumerable authors, may only list the first three, followed by et al. It is usually assumed that authors are named in order of their importance to the project. The problem with other kinds of ranking, such as alphabetical order or by prestige, is the likelihood of misinterpretation. The best rule is to list people in order of the significance of their contribution, however the group makes that determination.

Sometimes a single project evolves into several (it is hoped discrete) papers, and first authorship issues are resolved by rotating the order of the names on the different publications. Indeed, this is a common practice.

Perils of Prestige

Authorship or order of recognition should not rest on professional role or academic degree. No nurse should be forced to add the name of a more prestigious nurse to her independent work. Sometimes in the case of a dissertation, emotional blackmail is applied. My own bias is that faculty are paid to supervise dissertations and, like paid editors, should not be included as authors on publications stemming from a dissertation. There are other nurses who feel justified in supporting the counterargument that some chairmen become intensely involved in a student's work, providing enough of the leadership to merit inclusion. Indeed, there are some students who feel that attaching the name of a famous chair gives their work more prestige. I simply disagree with this perception, but, again, there is no iron-clad rule.

It is equally unfair when a more famous nurse is made first author over others if she truly did not merit that position on the list. Less experienced authors should bring issues of rank and merit to the attention of the whole group before such an inequity occurs.

SETTING THE GROUND RULES

The trick to collaborative writing is to do what any successful collaboration requires: Set the ground rules at the beginning of the project. That means deciding who will be responsible for what component of the project, including the final writing tasks. It means deciding in advance who is responsible for content, who will be recognized as authors, and in what sequence project contributions will relate to authors' ranking.

Unfortunately, there are few recognized rules concerning group authorship. There is a general consensus that everyone listed as an author of a work takes public responsibility for the content of the publication.

Problems occur when people forget this. Both unwarranted inclusions and exclusions can cause difficulties. Sometimes a person is identified as an author in what is anticipated to be a surprise honor. Such a favor turns out to be the opposite if the person disagrees with any aspect of the publication or if she simply finds the work of a quality to which she does not want her name attached. Disclaimers, if they must be published, prove a major embarrassment to the well-intentioned but misinformed party who included the person as author without first seeking permission.

In the opposite case, when someone who perceives herself to have been an integral part of the research is omitted as author, the scene is set for another unhappy outcome. I know of one case in which the nurse who did most of the work on a research project simply assumed she would be included in the subsequent publications. From her perspective, the project could not have occurred without her.

Unfortunately, her colleagues saw her merely as the person

who implemented their procedures. It never occurred to them that this nurse, who collected all the data and prepared it for their analysis, would feel that she had rights to authorship. Her disappointment and disaffection is reenacted in hundreds of projects yearly. This is why ground rules for inclusion and exclusion should be set and communicated in advance.

Nor can agreements concerning authorship go unreviewed during the course of a project. Some people will fail to keep their commitments; others will step in to replace them. New aspects may be added to the project; other aspects may be dropped. Initial agreements concerning who will and who will not be listed as authors may need to be reviewed at periodic intervals as the project advances.

Even in the best of circumstances it is difficult to weigh the importance of such various activities as generating the idea, designing the project, conducting the research, collecting the data, analyzing the data, and writing the manuscript. The importance of these and other elements will vary from project to project, making it impossible to develop iron-clad rules. Each group must make its own evaluation, develop its own sense of equity among the players.

In general it is agreed that anyone given author status has contributed significantly to the formulation, execution, or the analysis of the project and the writing up of the project. Authorship should certainly include those who have made substantial scientific contributions even if they were not the actual writers. All authors should review a final draft before a manuscript is submitted to any publisher. If any author cannot agree to the final draft, she has the right to remove her name at that time.

PRODUCTS OF GROUP WRITING

Group writing takes many forms. Sometimes a single article is the product with contributions by various writers blended together. In other instances, the product may be a book, a vehicle that allows different authors to contribute different chapters. Sometimes the Table of Contents will identify chapters by their various contributors. In other cases, group writing results in related articles appearing together or in sequential issues of a journal. For example, different authors might discuss competing therapies for a single clinical problem.

When an article is broken down into component assignments for several writers, there may be natural breaks in the content. A project might be divided into subsections such as the introduction, the project itself (the process), and the analysis of its effectiveness. In a more formalized research project, the areas might be separated into a literature review, the research methodology, the findings, and the analysis.

Coordinated writing may make sense when a group is dealing with:

- Closely related topics
- Serial projects where the conclusions of one phase lead to the next project
- Alternative approaches to the same clinical problem
- Alternative research methods applied to the same subject matter
- Separate studies within the context of a large research project
- Same subject matter content being organized for different audiences such as lay, professional, and paraprofessional

CREATING A UNIFIED WORK

In cases in which multiple writers participate in one book or article, there is a need to make the writing of whole cloth. Because no two writers have the same style, an article will appear disjointed if its components are not made homogeneous. Often this can be achieved by having one author responsible for the final version, creating an overall style and adapting the writing from all the contributors to that style.

Contributing writers need to understand the necessity for this finishing touch. An article will not work if some authors are too wedded to their own words. Groups should agree on a writing protocol before a project gets started; then there will not be unhappy surprises.

Books do not require the same degree of uniformity as an article, though it is still desirable to have some sense that things "fit" together. Sometimes a sense of uniformity can be achieved by setting an overall tone. It is disturbing to the reader, for example, if one chapter is "chatty," whereas the next sounds highly scholarly.

Uniformity also may be attained by having each writer address the same audience: what the *new* nurse practitioner needs to know, not just practitioner-related skills. This sort of approach, if carried out by every author, will give a sense of homogeneity to the manuscript.

Articles are too short to tolerate much deviation in style. Worse, even if the reader might not notice where one reader leaves off and another begins, an editor will. The irregularity in style may be enough to get an article rejected. It is just common sense to let one of the authors give an article the final requisite uniformity in style and syntax.

WHEN TOO MANY ARTICLES ARE PRODUCED IN A SINGLE PROJECT

Sometimes a problem arises because too many similar articles are offered to competitive journals. (In some of these instances, I have seen authors clearly guilty of plagiarizing themselves.) Editors become irate to discover an article submitted to their journal has appeared or is scheduled to appear elsewhere, only sightly changed in format, with nearly the same content.

The time is long since gone when nursing publications had more space than could be filled with articles. From an editor's perspective, it is important to bring to the reading nursing public as many different aspects of practice as possible. Where valuable space repeats essentially the same findings reported elsewhere, that opportunity is lost. Worse, the editor will remember the case and the involved authors when they submit another piece of work.

A simple rule for the new writer is that, however the words may vary, it is the same article if it presents the same information. and draws the same conclusions. A minimal overlap of facts is acceptable if the data are being used in different ways in the two articles.

PRIOR COMMITMENTS TO PUBLISH

Some collegial writing projects come about as the result of an idea that started in the mind of an editor—possibly a series of articles or an entire issue devoted to a single topic. Frequently invitations are sent out to those judged most capable of contributing to the series.

At other times, the pattern is reversed, and a collegial group proposes the notion of a collected work to an editor. Sometimes a group decides on such a proposal after a conference, when they realize the exceptional quality of the collected papers.

After-the-fact publication decisions are always more difficult, so writing/research groups should plan ahead. It is frustrating when an enthusiastic project group completes a major writing effort only to discover their subject matter does not interest any editor.

When potential editors or publishers are contacted in advance, they may be able to give advice as to how a project might be slanted to make the resultant book or article marketable. Often these suggestions can be built into the design of the project or into the writing.

It should be understood that initial agreement by an editor does not mean she is committed to publish an inferior work. If the work submitted is not up to standard, she has no such obligation.

ADVANTAGES OF COLLEGIAL WRITING

There are numerous advantages to group writing. First, it provides the writer with built-in criticism for her content and writing style. Having several people strengthens content because it provides a think-tank atmosphere. If, however, criticism is used the wrong way, it may become a leavening process, reducing everything to bland general consensus.

Where writing is based on the work of a research group, several benefits of participation flow to the young writer/researcher. Such a group lets experienced and inexperienced nurses and other health professionals work side by side. The contribution of the inexperienced nurse may be overseen by the more experienced researcher. Such a group allows participants to enhance each others' strengths and mitigate their weaknesses.

DISADVANTAGES OF COLLEGIAL WRITING

Just as there is an upside to group writing, there is an inevitable downside. Most of it has to do with human relations. Inevitably some persons will fail to carry through on their commitments; others will do more than their share. People will differ on everything from their interpretation of the findings to preferences concerning where the manuscript(s) should be published.

Often people miscalculate the need for coordination in group writing. The simplistic notion that every participant will simply write up "her part" and the parts will be added together, never works.

Someone must oversee the writing products just as someone needed to oversee the project itself.

SUMMARY

Group writing efforts may be rewarding, particularly if all plans and operating rules for the project are determined in advance. Writing with a group is a good way for a new writer to get assistance with the process. Conversely, group writing is not necessarily easier than working alone. Coordination efforts increase in proportion to the number of participants. And frustrations arise unless all show the same level of flexibility, good will, and cooperation.

Developing a sense of equity among group members is the key to both project management and to collegial writing. Group writing is an experience every writer should have sometime in her career. If nothing else, it will teach her about the discipline required in the group effort.

BIBLIOGRAPHY

Blancett, S. S. (1991). Who is entitled to authorship? *Nurse Educator*, *16*, 3.

Carty, B. (1994, April). The protean nature of the nurse informaticist. *Nursing & Health Care*, *15*, 174–177.

Nativio, D. G. (1993, Winter). Authorship. *Image*, *25*, 359.

Nehring, W., & Durham, J. D. (1986). Multiple authorship in nursing. *Journal of Nursing Education*, *11*, 15–18.

Sobralske, M. C. (1990). Writing in the disciplines: A nursing faculty perspective. *Nurse Educator*, *15*, 11–14.

Chapter 15

Writing From Research

O ften it is a research project that first stimulates a nurse to write for publication. Research projects provide the best stimuli: They not only give the writer something new and unique to say, but—if the research was well designed—they throw in validity as well. Further, they can be written up in the tried and true research formula, taking away the fear of writing. Indeed, one can say that in doing research of any kind one has an obligation to communicate one's findings.

We will not review the pros and cons of research designs here—there are enough books and experts to do that. Instead, we will assume that the research is well designed, and we will look at the task of getting it published.

TRADITIONAL RESEARCH REPORTING

When a nurse has completed a research project, she invariably wants to share it with others. This usually means she thinks first of writing it up for a research journal. There is no question that general research-based journals such as *Nursing Research, Western Journal of Nursing Research,* or *Research in Nursing and Health* carry a certain status.

Some of the specialty journals feature research reporting as well—*Journal of Clinical Nursing Research*, for example. In truth, most of us are vain enough to enjoy being published in vehicles of this sort now and then. It confirms that we are practicing at the peak of our scholarly capacities.

Additionally, there is a growing group of journals that mix research reports along with more traditional articles. *Heart and Lung* and *AORN* come to mind in the specialty category. Some general journals can be included in this group such as *Image* or the *Journal of Professional Nursing*. As nurses become more familiar with the research format, one can anticipate that more and more journals will provide this mix.

There is another advantage in using the research format, however, and that is the fact that traditional research reporting is the most stylized form of writing. It follows the same sequence as was used in the study itself: formulation of a research problem, literature review, selecting a methodology for inquiry, including sample decisions, instrument selection and design, and procedures; data collection and analysis; summary of findings and discussion of implications, including suggestions for application of study findings and suggestions for further research needed.

The presentation format is so structured that the writer's creativity has to show in the project, not in the article about it. Selection of articles for inclusion by editors of these journals has more to do with the nature of the study and its findings that with the writing itself. A well-designed study, carried out flawlessly, resulting in interesting knowledge: a sure recipe for publication. And for the new writer, that definitive structure may provide a great crutch.

Even better, the reporting structure mimics the structure of the research design itself. In other words, the article virtually writes itself. The trick is that one must do the research first. Research articles never start with the rumination, "Gee, I really ought to get something published."

Let us suppose the writer has completed a neat piece of research with interesting findings, or maybe even research further validating someone else's prior findings. Then it is time to study the research journals more carefully.

On careful inspection, the writer will discover that, even within the traditional format, there are subtle differences among journals. Some focus on method; others give method less attention, placing greater emphasis on implications. Others highlight findings and applications. The closer one's article comes to the journal preferences, the more likely one is to get an article accepted.

Some research journals allow a "preaching/teaching" element in which a writer can justify her method in detail. (Writers of qualitative research often feel the need to elaborate or justify their methods, even today.) Yet other journals start with the premise that their readers are skilled researchers. Editors and review boards of these journals will be turned off by harangues explaining and championing rather usual research methods.

The smart writer gets to know the journal's preferences before she writes a final draft. Or she may select her journal based on what part of her study really shines.

Sometimes a nurse does a research project expecting some exciting, controversial findings, only to be saddened when her study points to more mundane conclusions. If the writer thinks the findings are mundane, you can bet the editor will. The trick here is to provide an insightful section on implications—and select a journal that is interested in implications. Often all a researcher needs to do is think more deeply about her findings. Perhaps the findings are not nearly so mundane as she originally supposed.

FLAWS IN RESEARCH WRITING

I like to mark the advancement of nursing as a scholarly profession by the sorts of mistakes in research that get published over the years. From that perspective, I am pleased to report that the general quality of research writing in our journals keeps right on improving.

Seldom do we see the obvious mistakes any more. Findings are not extended to inappropriate populations; self-selected samples are not treated as if they were random; tools usually measure what they purport to measure. We have moved on to more sophisticated errors. I will only deal with two of them here—the ones I find most often.

Researcher With a Cause

Sometimes an inexperienced researcher is so attached to the results she wanted to get (as opposed to those she did get), that her article cannot break away from that commitment. Instead of considering the actual results, she encourages others to measure the phenomenon with greater refinement, to use more precise instruments—all in the hope that the results will contradict her own findings.

In effect, this writer is discounting her research. In my estimation, this is probably the second most common mistake in published research articles today. It is a mistake not made in the research journals whose editors are sophisticated in research design, incidentally. They simply will not publish an article with this error.

This mistake is often tied to that brilliant conclusion the researcher hoped to draw in the implications portion of her study. When a nurse has been anticipating writing implications for the opposite case, it may be difficult for her to switch gears. But switch gears, she must. Her discussion cannot be focused on finding the flaws in her study, showing why it must have been wrong. (If there was a whopper of a mistake in her methodology, we are not talking about publication anyway.)

Instead, if she has any faith in her own work, she must analyze the actual findings. We all know she should have been "neutral" to her findings in the first place, but we are talking about young researchers and writers here. The best advice I can give a writer who is disappointed in her findings is to get some space, then come back to them determined to search out the fascinating implications. With that attitude, she will write a good article.

Many an otherwise ordinary research report has been saved (and published) because of an insightful consideration of the study's implications—implications based on what was actually found, that is.

The most common error I find in research reports today has to do with a study's conceptual framework. Often the perceived framework has little or nothing to do with what was actually measured. I think this fault occurs because faculty demand that every dissertation have a conceptual framework, but they do not necessarily know what to do with it once the student produces one.

These mistakes, especially the latter one, represent a step up in research sophistication. I look forward to the day when it is difficult to find research reports with errors.

OTHER PUBLICATION OUTLETS FOR RESEARCH

Writers often forget that research can be reported in nonresearch journals too. Here the research is reported, but emphasis is shifted to findings, contextual factors of interest, applications, and implications. In other words, research can be adapted to the style used by any journal with just a little work. When an article based on research appears in a general journal, the researcher may not be able to devote much space to her research design. However, she certainly may indicate how the reader can get more information on that element if desired.

Sometimes a nurse decides that her findings are so important that they should be shared with practitioners who do not always read research journals. In this case, she may elect to convert a research report into the article format of a journal with a large subscription base for the sake of greater dispersion of the findings.

GETTING MILEAGE FROM A SINGLE RESEARCH PROJECT

As we mentioned in the last chapter, no editor is happy to find that an article she has printed or accepted for publication has been virtually duplicated in another journal. That does not mean that a research project must necessarily be restricted to one publication.

The researcher simply has to ask herself if there are distinct elements in her study that are worth separate reporting. Perhaps a complex measuring instrument has been designed and applied in collecting data. Is the tool one that would be useful to others for replication of this study or for other purposes? Perhaps the tool development or the substance of the tool itself merits a separate article. Chapter 16 provides suggestions for how tools may be presented in the literature.

Sometimes a critical literature review can become the basis for a scholarly article, providing that it goes beyond the "show-and-tell" stage, into a clever analysis of the "state of the art" for this subject matter. An analysis of the literature involves identifying trends spotted in the literature as well as identifying gaps or directions not taken by researchers. Further, it may be useful to discriminate between research on a subject and general articles about the subject based on nonresearched ideas. Nursing is often guilty of following certain values or traditions in spite of research to the contrary. Such a conflict is great grist for a publication. As we said earlier this sort of summary article is one of the hardest to sell, so it needs to be special.

If the study is a large one, it may have included several separate smaller studies within it, and one or more of these may merit a separate article. Much of the metaresearch or research using principles of triangulation rely on data from diverse sources, diverse methodologies.

Finally, the findings and implications may constitute a separate article is they are weighty. Or they may lend themselves to a discussion of how nursing practice should or can be altered in light of the study. Applications can be viewed through different practice lenses: One article might deal with how the findings impact on nursing management, whereas a second article might deal, instead, with how the individual nurse might alter her care practices.

Any of these tactics are fair game for extending the publications arising from a study, provided the articles really are different in content.

RESEARCHER'S RESPONSIBILITY TO REPORT

A final word about the responsibility of a researcher: Any researcher has a real responsibility to make her findings available to the larger nursing community. For purposes of this book, we have looked at the traditional method: getting the study published.

Failing that, the researcher still has an obligation to see that her study is accessible to other researchers. Many journals carry abbreviated research reports as do various computerized information services. Many nurses organizations (including many State Nurses' Associations) systematically survey their members in an attempt to collect information on all studies completed or in progress.

A writer who fails to get her study published may be discouraged and not seek out these alternate sources. Some nurses see submitting such briefs as "giving up." But any researcher has an obligation to inform the nursing public of her study by whatever means is available to her. Poster sessions at conferences and conventions are another opportunity.

Replication studies often suffer the fate of being difficult to market to journals, yet their importance cannot be overstated. Too often nursing makes changes in practice based on a single study, sometimes one based on a limited sample population or questionable methodologies. This, incidentally, is why every researcher must be willing to share her methods and tools with other researchers. Validation of findings (or lack thereof) is a normal part of the scientific process.

SUMMARY

Research reporting is both an obligation and, often, an easy way for the inexperienced writer to get a publication under her belt. The traditional research report, following the steps of the research process, provides an easy formula for writing.

Further, a researcher need not limit her publications to the traditional research journals. Any good research project can be discussed in various styles and adapted to the publication requirements of different journals.

BIBLIOGRAPHY

Beckstrand, J., & McBride, A. B. (1990). How to form a research interest group. *Nursing Outlook, 38*, 168–171.

Blancett, S. S. (1986). Getting your research published. *Journal of Nursing Administration, 16*, 4.

Carty, B. (1994). The protean nature of the nurse informaticist. *Nursing & Health Care, 15*, 174–177.

Cohen, M. Z., Knafl, K., & Dzurec, L. C. (1993). Grant writing for qualitative research. *Image, 25*, 151–156.

Flanagin, A. (1993, winter). Fraudulent publication. *Image, 25*, 359.

Tornquist, E. M. (1986). *From proposal to publication: An informal guide to writing about nursing research.* Menlo Park, CA: Addison-Wesley.

Tornquist, E. M., & Funk, S. G. (1990). How to write a research grant proposal. *Image, 22*, 44–51.

Chapter 16

Writing About Work Instruments

any nursing articles are written to explain a teaching, research, or measurement instrument, be it a patient instruction pamphlet, a research questionnaire, or perhaps a quality assessment tool. Other articles focus on the merits of products
that have been devised to meet certain medical and health requirements. Products range as far as the minds of their inventors, from
anatomically correct dolls to devices to help paraplegics hold spoon.

Whether the item be paper and pencil or a physical product,
we will call them all instruments for purposes of this discussion. The
successful presentation of an instrument in an article requires careful
planning; it is not an easy article to compose. Furthermore, many
decisions must be made prior to the writing.

OWNERSHIP OF THE INSTRUMENT

The first question is one of ownership of the instrument itself. This
must be settled before considering who has the right to write about
it. Even if a nurse has found an instrument that works miracles,
she cannot display it in writing without the owner's permission.

Sometimes a nurse mistakenly assumes that the instrument is hers if she developed it. That simply is not the case if its creation was part of her job and the tool is an operating document or in-use instrument of the institution.

Suppose, for example, that a nurse in quality management designed a discharge planning form that is now used on the various nursing units of her hospital. Assume she was not specifically assigned to create that particular tool. Still, creating the form was within the scope of her job description. Most would rightly judge the tool to be the property of the institution, not the nurse.

If the tool was developed as part of the nurse's work assignment, on work time, then—in the absence of other prior agreements—the ownership of the instrument belongs to the institution. But not all cases are as obvious as this one.

And there are instances when a tool developed by a nurse employed in an institution can be judged to be the sole property of the nurse who created it. Let us suppose a nurse created a unique teaching tool, a game board that instructs patients on how to calculate cholesterol levels in foods, for example. Suppose that the creation, design, and testing of the tool occurred on her own time, not during work hours, albeit that the incentive for creating the tool arose because of the patient group under her care. Suppose further that she assumed the cost of producing the instrument. And when and if she used the tool in her place of employment, those who played the game derived a benefit from it.

Usually it is assumed that creative tools such as the cholesterol counting game board belong to their creator—assuming that the nurse was not hired for the specific purpose of designing such a tool and assuming that the tool was not created on company time. Many games, certain computer software programs, as well as products—children's story books or toys designed for therapeutic purposes, for example—come under this heading: items the creation of which exceeds the scope and vision of normal employment.

Nevertheless, there have been cases in which ownership of creative products has been challenged. Because there have been disputes over ownership, and because the circumstances surrounding an instrument's creation may be blurred, the nurse should consider her legal rights carefully. If the nurse is creating a tool for which she envisions retaining sole property rights, she would be wise to reach a prior understanding with her employer in writing.

PERMISSIONS AND ACKNOWLEDGMENTS

In cases in which an institution is the owner of a tool, an author must first acquire a release from the institution before exhibiting the instrument, in whole or in part, in the public press. An author who wishes to write about such a tool must seek permission from the highest corporate nurse executive (unless the institution has a different policy) before releasing information about the tool in the literature, lay or professional.

If the tool is a good one, permission often will be given because it is to the institution's credit to display its effective tools. The institution may be pleased to share the instrument with others so that they may benefit from its application. In that case, the article may display the entire instrument and indicate that it may be reproduced without permission.

Conversely, if an institution itself plans to market the instrument, administrators may be less than pleased to find the tool displayed in its entirety in a journal, even if the article indicates that the tool may not be further reproduced. To ensure that a tool is not copied, some articles describe an instrument but do not display it except for a few illustrative segments. The article then indicates how readers may purchase the complete tool. In this way an article can serve as an excellent means of advertising while still protecting the owner's rights.

If the writer is the creator and owner of the tool, one obstacle is eliminated. Unless the article states otherwise, an editor will assume that is the case.

The writer should be warned that editors are sensitive to commercial situations of this sort and will seldom publish an article whose only purpose is to sell an instrument or service of an institution. The article must, in itself and separate from the tool, have something to offer the reader before an editor will consider it.

Sometimes the difference between creation and ownership of a tool can be resolved by the following procedure: The creator authors a paper describing the instrument, hence getting recognition for her instrument. In the same article, the institution (the owner) is recognized and acknowledged as the place where the tool was developed and tested. Acknowledgment in this form is often a satisfactory payoff for the institution.

What about the case in which the author writes about a useful tool created by another party? This should happen only when all parties are in agreement and the creator of the tool is acknowledged in the article.

The rights of the creator cannot be usurped by the writer. Sometimes the resolution involves making the creator a coauthor of the paper. Negotiation with the creator of the instrument should determine both authorship of the article and acknowledgement credits. See Chapter 14 for some of the issues involved in such a situation.

PURPOSES SERVED BY WRITING ABOUT AN INSTRUMENT

For purposes of this discussion we are more interested in the article to be written than in the creation of a particular instrument itself. Many different purposes may be served by an article featuring a tool, and the writer should have one—and only one—in mind when writing the article. Typical purposes might be:

- To share a useful tool with other nursing organizations. In this case the article will present the entire tool, describe the procedures used to implement it, and explain its purpose and value.

- To make available a valuable tool that other nursing organizations may wish to purchase. The difference between this and the first sort of article is the addition of financial incentive. When this is the intention, the tool should be protected by being under copyright or patent law as they apply.
- To advocate that institutions create tools of this sort, to do this task, to achieve these objectives. In this case the specific tool is not as important as is the unique purpose it serves. Here the tool simply becomes an illustration of how such a purpose might be executed.
- To describe the unique process that leads to the creation of such a tool. Where numerous groups or individuals with potentially conflicting motives had to be drawn together to produce the tool, the process itself becomes fascinating reading. In this case, the process is the message rather than the particular content of the tool itself.

If the same article attempts to serve more than one of these purposes, it is likely to become diffuse and undirected. In each case, the article must stand on its own, even, or one might say especially, if it concerns an interesting instrument.

WRITING THE ARTICLE

There are often unsuspected difficulties in writing about an instrument. If the instrument is displayed in its entirety, the author may have difficulty figuring what else to say besides, "Here it is." If the instrument is displayed only in selected examples, it may be difficult to describe accurately its total content and purpose.

Where the tool is displayed in its entirety, accompanying content should not repeat the obvious; in other words, do not repeat in the explanation things already said in the tool. The author can talk about the purpose of the tool, the variables it addresses, how the tool was validated, how it was accepted by those using it, what was achieved with the data collected in its use.

For example, in a performance appraisal instrument designed to rate nurses in intensive care units, the article might discuss how the major categories were derived, how many nurses were evaluated using the tool, how they felt about the tool's efficacy.

If there were interesting problems in the tool's creation, those might be included. For example, I know of one instance when a patient teaching tool was translated into a second language by a translator whose choice of words, while not inaccurate, was too sophisticated to be understood in the poorly educated non–English-speaking community where the tool was to be used. It was that nurse's first lesson in the subtleties of translation.

The worst mistake an author can make when discussing a tool presented in its entirety, is to go down the list, item by item, discussing each entry. Quite simply, this makes a boring article with little chance of acceptance for publication.

Conversely, where only examples of selected items of the tool are offered, it is important that the reader get a grasp of the total instrument even though she won't see each item. Sometimes the author who created a tool is too close to it to recognize when her article fails to describe it adequately. In this case, it is a good idea to have the article evaluated by a colleague. The reader should come away with a sense of the sort of items that would appear in the sections not illustrated.

Where the article is meant to describe the process of deriving a tool, there are different traps. No reader wants to know that ten people met around a table on the fifth of the month in the school of nursing's cafeteria. An article that reads like the minutes of the meeting has little chance of publication, no matter how dear those details are to the writer.

The process should be described in terms of the issues and objectives of the players. What incentives were necessary to gain this approval? Why was that cooperation essential? How were recalcitrant but essential members won over? How were others who would later use the tool made to feel part of the process? How were groups trained to use the tool? Stick to the issues, the arguments, the obstructions, and the tactics. The writer should not give a schedule of meetings and their agendas, details that only have meaning to the institution where the work was accomplished.

SUMMARY

Nurses often enjoy writing about tools they have created. The topic is near to their hearts and they know their tools better than anyone else does. Furthermore, articles about instruments can be valuable and concrete resources for others. Authors should beware, however, of the dual set of problems involved in such articles: problems of ownership and entitlement related to both the instrument itself and the article.

With careful planning and necessary agreements among all parties involved, an article about an instrument can be successful and rewarding. Further, it can provide a real service for the nursing community.

Appendices

Appendix A

*LIST OF NURSING JOURNALS (PARTIAL)**

AACN CLINICAL ISSUES IN CRITICAL CARE NURSING
American Association of Critical Care Nurses
Philadelphia, PA

AANA JOURNAL
American Association of Nurse Anesthetists
Chicago, IL

AAOHN JOURNAL
(Occupational Health Nursing)
Charles B. Slack
Thorofare, NJ

ALTERNATIVE HEALTH PRACTITIONER
Springer Publishing Compnay
New York, NY

*List does not include state or university publications, nor foreign entries
except for some common journals of Great Britain and Canada.

AMERICAN JOURNAL OF NURSING
American Journal of Nursing Company
New York, NY

AMERICAN NURSE (newspaper)
American Nurses Association
Washington, DC

ANNA JOURNAL
American Nephrology Nurses Association
Pitman, NJ

ADVANCES IN NURSING SCIENCE
Aspen Systems Corp.
Germantown, MD

AORN JOURNAL
Association of Operating Room Nurses
Denver, CO

APPLIED NURSING RESEARCH
W. B. Saunders
Philadelphia, PA

ARCHIVES OF PSYCHIATRIC NURSING
Grune and Stratton
Orlando, FL

ASPEN ADVISOR FOR NURSE EXECUTIVES
Aspen Publishers
Rockville, MD

CANADIAN CRITICAL CARE NURSING JOURNAL
Society of Critical Care Nurses of Canada
Toronto, Canada

CANADIAN JOURNAL OF CARDIOVASCULAR NURSING
Canadian Council of Cardiovascular Nurses of the
Heart and Stroke Foundation of Canada
Ottawa, Canada

CANADIAN JOURNAL OF NURSING ADMINISTRATION
Health Media
Toronto, Canada

CANADIAN JOURNAL OF NURSING RESEARCH
School of Nursing, McGill University
Montreal, Canada

CANADIAN JOURNAL OF PSYCHIATRIC NURSING
Psychiatric Nurses Association of Canada
New Westminster, Canada

CANADIAN NURSE
Canadian Nurses Association
Ottawa, Canada

CANADIAN OPERATING ROOM NURSING JOURNAL
Operating Room Nurses of Canada
Health Media
Ontario, Canada

CANCER NURSING
Raven Press
New York, NY

CARDIOVASCULAR NURSING
American Hearth Association
New York, NY

CLINICAL ISSUES IN OBSTETRICS, GYNECOLOGIC AND NEO-
NATAL NURSING
Organization for Obstetric, Gynecologic and Neonatal Nurses
J. B. Lippincott
Philadelphia, PA

CLINICAL NURSE SPECIALIST
Williams & Wilkins
Baltimore, MD

CLINICAL NURSING RESEARCH
Sage Publications
Newbury Park, CA

COMPUTERS IN NURSING
J. B. Lippincott
Philadelphia, PA

CONA JOURNAL
Canadian Orthopaedic Nurses Association
Toronto, Canada

CRITICAL CARE NURSING CLINICS OF NORTH AMERICA
W. B. Saunders
Philadelphia, PA

CRITICAL CARE NURSING QUARTERLY
Aspen Publishers
Frederick, MD

CRNA: THE JOURNAL FOR NURSE ANESTHETIST
W. B. Saunders
Philadelphia, PA

DIMENSIONS OF CRITICAL CARE NURSING
J. B. Lippincott
Philadelphia, PA

GASTROENTEROLOGY NURSING
Society of Gastroenterology Nurses and Associates
Williams & Wilkins
Baltimore, MD

GERIATRIC NURSING
American Journal of Nursing Company
New York, NY

HEALTH PROGRESS
Catholic Health Association of the United States
St. Louis, MO

HEART AND LUNG: THE JOURNAL OF CRITICAL CARE
Mosby-Year Book
St. Louis, MO

HOLISTIC NURSING PRACTICE
Aspen Publishers
Frederick, MD

HOME HEALTH CARE NURSE
American Association of Occupational Health Nurses
J. B. Lippincott
Philadelphia, PA

HOSPITAL & HEALTH SERVICES ADMINISTRATION
Foundation of the Americal College of Healthcare Executives
Chicago, IL

IMAGE—THE JOURNAL OF NURSING SCHOLARSHIP
Sigma Theta Tau, National Honor Society of Nursing
Indianapolis, IN

IMPRINT
National Student Nurses Association
New York, NY

INTERNATIONAL JOURNAL OF NURSING STUDIES
Pergamon Press
Oxford, Great Britain

INTERNATIONAL NURSING REVIEW
International Council of Nurses
Geneva, Switzerland

ISSUES IN COMPREHENSIVE PEDIATRIC NURSING
Hemisphere Publishing
New York, NY

ISSUES IN MENTAL HEALTH NURSING
Hemisphere Publishing
New York, NY

JOURNAL OF ADVANCED NURSING
Blackwell Scientific Publications
Oxford, Great Britain

JOURNAL OF THE AMERICAN ACADEMY OF
NURSE PRACTITIONERS
American Academy of Nurse Practitioners
Philadelphia, PA

JOURNAL OF THE ASSOCIATION OF NURSES IN AIDS CARE
Nursecom Inc. Publishers
Philadelphia, PA

JOURNAL CANNT
Canadian Association of Nephrology Nurses and Technicians
Pembroke, Canada

JOURNAL OF CARDIOVASCULAR NURSING
Aspen Publishers
Frederick, MD

JOURNAL OF CASE MANAGEMENT
Springer Publishing Company
New York, NY

JOURNAL OF CHILD AND ADOLESCENT PSYCHIATRIC AND
MENTAL HEALTH NURSING
J. B. Lippincott
Philadelphia, PA

JOURNAL OF COMMUNITY HEALTH NURSING
Lawrence Erlbaum Associates
Hillsdale, NJ

JOURNAL OF CONTINUING EDUCATION IN NURSING
Charles B. Slack
Thorofare, NJ

JOURNAL OF EMERGENCY NURSING
Mosby-Year Book
St. Louis, MO

JOURNAL OF GERONTOLOGICAL NURSING
Charles B. Slack
Thorofare, NJ

JOURNAL OF HOLISTIC NURSING
American Holistic Nurses Association
Springfield, MO

JOURNAL OF INTRAVENOUS NURSING
J. B. Lippincott
Hagerstown, MD

JOURNAL OF LONG TERM CARE ADMINISTRATION
American College of Nursing Home Administration
Silver Spring, MD

JOURNAL OF LONG-TERM HOME HEALTH CARE
Springer Publishing Company
New York, NY

JOURNAL OF NATIONAL BLACK NURSES ASSOCIATION
National Black Nurses Association
Boston, MA

JOURNAL OF NEUROSCIENCE NURSING
American Association of Neuroscience Nurses
Park Ridge, IL

JOURNAL OF NURSE-MIDWIFERY
American College of Nurse-Midwives
Elsevier
New York, NY

JOURNAL OF NURSING ADMINISTRATION
J. B. Lippincott
Philadelphia, PA

JOURNAL OF NURSING CARE QUALITY
Aspen Publishers
Frederick, MD

JOURNAL OF NURSING EDUCATION
Charles B. Slack
Thorofare, NJ

JOURNAL OF NURSING MEASUREMENT
Springer Publishing Company
New York, NY

JOURNAL OF OPHTHALMIC NURSING AND TECHNOLOGY
Charles B. Slack
Thorofare, NJ

JOURNAL OF PEDIATRIC HEALTH CARE
C. V. Mosby
St. Louis, MO

JOURNAL OF PEDIATRIC NURSING
W. B. Saunders
Philadelphia, PA

JOURNAL OF PEDIATRIC ONCOLOGY NURSING
Association of Pediatric Oncology Nurses
W. B. Saunders
Philadelphia, PA

JOURNAL OF PERINATAL AND NEONATAL NURSING
Aspen Publishers
Frederick, MD

JOURNAL OF POST ANESTHESIA NURSING
Grune and Stratton
Orlando, FL

JOURNAL OF PRACTICAL NURSING
National Association for Practical Nurse Education and Service
St. Louis, MO

JOURNAL OF PROFESSIONAL NURSING
American Association of Colleges of Nursing
W. B. Saunders
Philadelphia, PA

JOURNAL OF PSYCHOSOCIAL NURSING AND MENTAL HEALTH
SERVICES
Charles B. Slack
Thorofare, NJ

JOURNAL/SOCIETY OF OTORHINOLARYNGOLOGY AND HEAD-
NECK NURSES
Society of Otorhinolaryngology and Head-Neck Nurses
Warren, OH

JOURNAL OF TRANSCULTURAL NURSING
Transcultural Nursing Society
Memphis College of Nursing, University of Tennessee
Memphis, TN

JOURNAL OF UROLOGICAL NURSING
International Urological Sciences
Long Valley, NY

JOURNAL OF WOUND, OSTOMY, AND CONTINENCE NURSING
Wound, Ostomy, and Continence Nurses Society
C. V. Mosby
St. Louis, MO

LAW, MEDICINE AND HEALTH CARE
American Society of Law and Medicine
Boston, MA

MCN: AMERICAN JOURNAL OF MATERNAL CHILD NURSING
American Journal of Nursing Company
New York, NY

NAACOG CLINICAL ISSUES IN PERINATAL AND WOMENS
HEALTH NURSING
Nurses Association of the American Colleges of Obstetricians and
Gynecologists
Philadelphia, PA

NAACOG NEWLETTER
Nurses Association of the American Colleges of Obstetricians and
Gynecologists
Washington, DC

NEONATAL NETWORK
National Association of Neonatal Nurses
San Francisco, CA

NURSE ANESTHESIA
Appleton and Lange
East Norwalk, CT

NURSE EDUCATOR
J. B. Lippincott
Philadelphia, PA

NURSE EXECUTIVE
American Organization of Nurse Executives
Chicago, IL

NURSE MANAGERS BOOKSHELF
Williams & Wilkins
Baltimore, MD

THE NURSE PRACTITIONER: THE AMERICAN JOURNAL OF PRIMARY HEALTH CARE
Uniformed Nurse Practitioner Association
Elsevier Science, Inc., NY

NURSING (94, 95, ETC.)
Springhouse
Springhouse, PA

NURSING ADMINISTRATION QUARTERLY
Aspen Systems
Germantown, MD

NURSING CLINICS OF NORTH AMERICA
W. B. Saunders
Philadelphia, PA

NURSING DIAGNOSIS
North American Nursing Diagnosis Association
J. B. Lippincott
Philadelphia, PA

NURSING ECONOMICS
Anthony J. Jannetti
Pitman, NJ

NURSING FORUM
Nursecom Inc.
Philadelphia, PA

NURSING & HEALTH CARE
National League for Nursing
New York, NY

NURSING LEADERSHIP FORUM
Springer Publishing Company
New York, NY

NURSING MANAGEMENT
SN Publications
Chicago, IL

NURSING OUTLOOK
Mosby Yearbook
St. Louis, MO

NURSING RESEARCH
American Journal of Nursing Company
New York, NY

NURSING SCIENCE QUARTERLY
Chestnut House Publishers
Pittsburgh, PA

NURSING TIMES
Macmillan Journals
London, Great Britain

NURSING YEARBOOK
Springhouse Corporation
Springhouse, PA

OCCUPATIONAL HEALTH AND SAFETY
Stevens Publishing
Waco, TX

OFFICE NURSE
J and T Publishing
Montvale, NJ

ONCOLOGY NURSING FORUM
Oncology Nursing Society
New York, NY

PUBLIC HEALTH NURSING
Blackwell Scientific Publications
Boston, MA

REGAN REPORT ON NURSING LAW
Medica Press
Providence, RI

REGISTERED NURSE
BCS Communications
Toronto, Canada

REHABILITATION NURSING
Association of Rehabilitation Nursing
Evanston, IL

RESEARCH IN NURSING AND HEALTH
Wiley
New York, NY

RN
Medical Economics
Oradel, NJ

RNAO NEWS
Registered Nurses Association of Ontario
Toronto, Canada

ROGERIAN NURSING SCIENCE NEWS
Society of Rogerian Scholars
New York, NY

SCHOLARLY INQUIRY FOR NURSING PRACTICE
Springer Publishing Company
New York, NY

SCI NURSING
American Association of Spinal Cord Injury Nurses
New York, NY

SEMINARS IN ONCOLOGY NURSING
W. B. Saunders
Philadelphia, PA

SOCIETY FOR NURSING HISTORY GAZETTE
Society for Nursing History
New York, NY

SPVN
Society for Peripheral Vascular Nursing
Norwood, MA

TODAYS OR NURSE
Charles B. Slack
Thorofare, NJ

UROLOGIC NURSING
American Urological Association Allied
Portland, OR

WESTERN JOURNAL OF NURSING RESEARCH
Sage Publications
Beverly Hills, CA

WHO AIDS SERIES
World Health Organization/International Council of Nursing
Geneva, Switzerland

Appendix B

LIST OF PUBLISHERS OF NURSING BOOKS (PARTIAL)*

Addison-Wesley Publishing Company
Menlo Park, CA

American Journal of Nursing Company
New York, NY

American Nurses Association
Washington, DC

Appleton & Lange
Norwalk, CT

Aspen Publishers
Rockville, MD

Blackwell Scientific Publications
Boston, MA

*List is partial and does not include specialty organizations or university presses.

Charles B. Slack
Thorofare, NJ

F. A. Davis Company
Philadelphia, PA

Delmar Publishers Inc.
Albany, NY

Grune & Stratton
New York, NY

J. B. Lippincott Company
Philadelphia, PA

John Wiley and Sons, Inc.
New York, NY

Jones and Bartlett Publishers
Boston, MA

Mosby-Year Book, Inc.
St. Louis, MO

National League for Nursing
New York, NY

Reston
Reston, VA

Sage Publications
Newbury Park, CA

Springer Publishing Company
New York, NY

Springhouse
Springhouse, PA

W. B. Saunders Company
Philadelphia, PA

Williams & Wilkins Company
Baltimore, MD

Appendix C

ADDITIONAL WRITING RESOURCES

Author & Editor. Hall Johnson Communications, 9737 W. Ohio Avenue, Lakewood, CO 80226.

Blank, J. J., & McElmurry, B. J. (1988). A profile of nursing journal editors. *Nursing Outlook, 36,* 179–181.

Gay, J. T., Edgil, A. E., & Rozmus, C. (1989). Nursing journals read and assigned most often in doctoral programs. *Image, 21,* 246–248.

Graves, J. R. (1993). Data versus information versus knowledge. *Reflections, 19,* 4–5.

Jordan, L. (Ed.). (1976). *The New York Times manual of style and usage.* New York: The New York Times Book Co.

Literary Market Place (Annual). New York: Bowker.

Miller, C., & Swift, K. (1988). *The handbook of nonsexist writing.* New York: Harper & Row.

Roget, P. M., enlarged by Roget, J. L., & Roget, S. R. (1980). *Roget's thesaurus of synonyms and antonyms.* New York: Modern Promotions.

Sinclair, V. G. (1987). Literature searches by computer. *Image, 19,* 35–37.

Sparks, S. M. Electronic networking for nurses. *Image, 25*, 245–248.

Strunk, W. J., & White, E. B. (1979). *The elements of style* (3rd ed.). New York: MacMillan Publishing Co.

Swanson, E., & McCloskey, J. (1986). Publishing opportunities for nurses. *Nursing Outlook*, 34, 227–235.

Writer's Market. (Annual). Cincinnati, OH: Writer's Digest Books.

Index

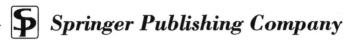 **Springer Publishing Company**

THE NURSE AS GROUP LEADER
3rd Edition

Carolyn Chambers Clark,
EdD, RN, ARNP, FAAN

This book is useful in a wide range of settings—from teaching groups to supportive or therapeutic groups to committee work with other health care providers. Simulated exercises in the book provide opportunity for practice. New to this edition are chapters on working with the elderly in groups, and on working with groups with specific problems, such as eating disorders, rape, or depression.

Contents:

Introduction to Group Work • Basic Group Concepts and Process • Working to Achieve Group Goals • Special Group Problems • Beginning, Guiding, and Terminating the Group • Supervision of Group Leaders and Co-leadership • Behavioral Approaches for Group Leaders • Recording • Groups for the Older Adult • Working With Focal Groups • When the Organization is the Group • When the Community is the Group

Springer Series : Teaching of Nursing
1994 304pp 0-8261-2333-3 softcover

536 Broadway, New York, NY 10012-3955 • (212) 431-4370 • Fax (212) 941-7842

Springer Publishing Company

NURSE-PHYSICIAN COLLABORATION
Care of Adults and the Elderly

Eugenia L. Siegler, MD, and
Fay W. Whitney, PhD, RN, FAAN, Editors

Foreword by Joan Lynaugh and Barbara Bates

Written by an RN-MD team, this book describes the current barriers to effective collaboration between nurses and physicians and suggests how to overcome them. Six successful examples of collaborative practice in a variety of settings are described. Specific guidelines for teaching collaborative skills to both physicians and nurses are outlined at length. Today's health care trends are toward expanded use of nurse practitioners and other nurses with advanced training. In these circumstances, successful collaboration can mean better health care delivery for all.

Contents:

Part I. Background. What is Collaboration? • Education of Physicians and Nurses • Social and Economic Barriers to Collaborative Practice

Part II. Examples of Collaborative Practices. Ambulatory Care • The Nursing Home • Home Care • The Post-Stroke Consultation Service • The Intensive Care Unit • Continuity of Care

Part III. Education. Teaching Collaboration to Nursing and Medical Undergraduates • Teaching Collaborative Skills to Nurse Practitioner Students.

Part IV. Research. Instruments for Studying Collaboration. • Collaborative Practice: Research Question. • Conclusion: Collaboration Past and Future

Springer Series: Advance Nursing Practice
1994 280pp (est.) 0-8261-8500-2 hardcover

536 Broadway, New York, NY 10012-3955 • (212) 431-4370 • Fax (212) 941-7842

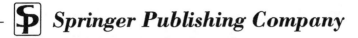

Springer Publishing Company

NURSES, NURSE PRACTITIONERS
Evolution to Advanced Practice
New Edition

Mathy D. Mezey, RN, EdD, FAAN and
Diane O. McGivern, RN, PhD, FAAN, Editors

This comprehensive guide to advanced practice nursing covers practical and conceptual issues with equal authority. It examines the evolution of nurses practitioners and other nurse specialists into the new advanced practice nursing role, and discusses its implications for the nursing profession and the health care system.

"...All the pertinent, complex, and complicated challenges facing nursing and nurse practitioners are explored by authors whose sterling reputations as experts make this section a fascinating compendium that every nurse practitioner and others will find indispensable for learning about the past, present, and future of the field."
—Loretta C. Ford, RN, EdD, FAAN

Partial Contents:

Part I. Philosophical, Historical, Educational, and Research Perspectives. The Evolution of Primary Care Practice, *D.O. McGivern* • Preparation for Advanced Practice, *M. Mezey* • Research in Support of Nurse Practitioners, *C.M. Freund* • Philosophical and Historical Bases of Primary Care Nursing, *E.D. Baer* **Part II: The Practice Arena.** Nurse Midwifery and Primary Health Care for Women, *J.E. Thompson* • Meeting the Health Care Needs of Older Adults, *N.E. Strumpf & G. Paier* • Nursing Centers: The New Arena for Advance Nursing Practice, *E. Sullivan, et al.* **Part III: Legislation, Law Reimbursement and Policy.** State Nurse Practice Acts, *B. Bullough* • Third-Party Reimbursement for Services of Nurses in Advanced Practice: Obtaining Payment for Your Services, *P. Mittelstadt*

Springer Series: Advanced Practice Nursing
1993   400pp   0-8261-7770-7   hardcover

536 Broadway, New York, NY 10012-3955 • (212) 431-4370 • Fax (212) 941-7842

Springer Publishing Company

JOURNAL

NURSING LEADERSHIP FORUM

Barbara Stevens Barnum, RN, PhD, FAAN, Editor

Advisory Board: Sarah Archer, Sheila Burke, Colleen Conway-Welch, Donna Diers, Rosemary Donley, Rhetaugh Dumas, Jerry Durham, Joyce Fitzpatrick, Maryann Fralic, Terry Fulmer, Karen Kowalski, Ruth Watson Lubic, Angela McBride, Carol Romano, Virginia Saba, Florence Selder, Hilda Steppe, Ora Strickland, Margretta Styles, Peter Ungvarski, Duane Walker, Gail Weissman

Nursing Leadership Forum is a quarterly refereed journal designed for the professional nurse who performs any of the diverse forms of leadership demanded of nurses—leadership with patients and families, nursing staff, health care institutions, or the larger community. Within this broad context, the journal explores the ethics, values, and theories underlying the exercise of nursing leadership, as well as innovative ideas for leadership effectiveness.

Sample Contents:

- Life Transition Theory: It Works for the Unemployed Nurse Executive as Well as for Patients, *E. Barba & F. Selder*
- Shifting Paradigms: An Approach to Teaching in an Era of Rapid Change, *J. P. Flynn*
- Nursing Leadership with the Pen: Two Peas in a Pod, *H. Forman*
- Preparing the Nurse Executive of the Future, *H. Feldman*
- Spirituality in Nursing: Everything Old is New Again, *B.S. Barnum*

ISSN 1076-1632 (4 issues annually)

536 Broadway, New York, NY 10012-3955 • (212) 431-4370 • Fax (212) 941-7842